BARIATRIC DIET

COOKBOOK

A Comprehensive Guide to Eating Well and Losing Weight with Delicious and Nutritious Recipes to Help You Achieve Your Weight Loss Goals

MILTON B. GRAHAM

CONTENTS

INTRODUCTION

You should be congratulated for taking the first step in maintaining a healthy lifestyle. The choice to have bariatric surgery may significantly alter one's life, and it is essential to be well-prepared for the considerable changes that will accompany this decision. When it comes to your post-surgical journey, your food is one of the most crucial factors to consider. Your success must adhere to a bariatric diet plan, both in terms of reaching your weight reduction goals and maintaining your general health.

For the duration of your voyage, this cookbook is intended to serve as both a guide and a companion. Not only will we provide you with all the facts you need to comprehend the bariatric diet, but we will also present you with meals that are both enjoyable and healthy to assist you in remaining on track.

DO YOU KNOW WHAT THE BARIATRIC DIET IS?

People who have had weight-loss surgery are the target audience for the bariatric diet, which is a specialized eating plan devised just for them. These are the guiding concepts that it is founded on:

Small portions: Because of the tiny size of your stomach after surgery, you will need to consume meals that are smaller and more often spaced apart.

High protein: Protein is crucial for healing and recuperation; hence, the bariatric diet prioritizes protein-rich meals.

Low fat: Fatty foods might be difficult to digest following surgery; therefore, the bariatric diet reduces fat intake.

Low sugar: Sugar may produce dumping syndrome, a collection of painful sensations that might occur after consuming specific meals.

Enough fluids: stay It is crucial to keep hydrated following surgery; thus, the bariatric diet encourages drinking enough water and other fluids.

The advantages of the bariatric diet

Following the bariatric diet may bring various advantages, including:

Weight loss: The bariatric diet is meant to help you lose weight and keep it off.

Improved health: The bariatric diet may help improve your overall health by lowering your risk of chronic illnesses such as heart disease, diabetes, and certain kinds of cancer.

Increased energy: Eating a balanced diet might give you more energy and enhance your mood.

Better quality of life: Following the bariatric diet may help you live a more active and satisfying life.

WHAT YOU WILL DISCOVER IN THIS COOKBOOK

This cookbook is filled with information and recipes to help you make the most of your bariatric diet. Here's a sneak peek at what you'll find:

A complete review of the bariatric diet: We'll cover all you need to know about the many stages of the diet, what to eat and what to avoid, and recommendations for making good choices.

Delicious and healthy dishes: We've included over 100 recipes for breakfast, lunch, supper, snacks, and desserts. All of the dishes are bariatric-friendly and crafted using fresh, healthy ingredients.

Meal planning: We've also provided example meal plans to help you get started. These meal plans are based on the bariatric diet requirements and offer a range of healthy alternatives.

Ideas and techniques: We'll provide some useful ideas and tactics for remaining on track with your diet, controlling cravings, and avoiding common bariatric surgery problems.

We recognize that following a new diet may be tough, but we're here to support you every step of the way. This cookbook is your reference for all you need to know about the bariatric diet. With our recipes, suggestions, and support, you can reach your weight reduction goals and live a better, happier life.

AN OVERVIEW OF BARIATRIC SURGERY

Bariatric surgery, commonly known as weight-loss surgery, is a collection of treatments that modify the digestive system to help patients with obesity lose weight and improve their health. It is considered a last choice when previous measures of weight reduction, such as diet and exercise, have failed.

Who is eligible for bariatric surgery?

Bariatric surgery is often indicated for those with a body mass index (BMI) of 40 or higher or those with a BMI of 35 or higher who have one or more weight-related health issues, such as:

- Type 2 diabetes
- Heart disease
- Sleep apnea

- High blood pressure
- Severe acid reflux
- Non-alcoholic fatty liver disease

TYPES OF BARIATRIC SURGERY

Gastric bypass: This is the most prevalent kind of bariatric surgery. In this operation, the surgeon constructs a tiny pouch in the stomach and then skips most of the small intestine. This restricts the quantity of food you can consume and the amount of nutrients your body absorbs.

Sleeve gastrostomy: In this treatment, the surgeon eliminates around 80% of the stomach, leaving a long, tube-shaped stomach pouch. This decreases the quantity of food you can consume and makes you feel full sooner.

Adjustable gastric band: This is a laparoscopic technique that includes inserting an adjustable band around the upper region of the stomach. The band may be tightened or relaxed over time to manage the quantity of food that can pass through the stomach.

Risks and advantages of bariatric surgery

Infection   Leakage from the operative site

Bleeding   Nutritional deficiencies

Dumping syndrome, which is a combination of symptoms that may develop after consuming particular foods

However, the advantages of bariatric surgery frequently exceed the concerns. Studies have shown that bariatric surgery may lead to considerable weight reduction, improved health, and a higher quality of life.

What to anticipate after bariatric surgery?

After bariatric surgery, you will need to follow a rigorous diet and activity regimen to help you lose weight and keep it off. You will also need to take frequent vitamin and mineral supplements to avoid nutritional deficits.

Bariatric surgery is a life-changing choice. It is crucial to thoroughly assess the dangers and advantages before determining whether it is good for you.

UNDERSTANDING THE BARIATRIC DIET

A bariatric diet is a customized eating regimen created for persons who have had bariatric surgery, such as gastric bypass or gastric sleeve surgery. These procedures are done to assist persons with extreme obesity in losing weight by lowering the size of the stomach and, in some circumstances, modifying the digestive process.

The major aims of a bariatric diet are to facilitate weight reduction, guarantee good recovery following surgery, and supply critical nutrients while restricting the consumption of calories and particular kinds of foods. The diet normally develops through multiple phases, beginning with a liquid or pureed diet and progressively graduating to solid meals.

Clear Liquid Phase

- ➢ Begins shortly after surgery and generally lasts for the first several days.
- ➢ Involves transparent liquids such as water, broth, sugar-free gelatin, and clear fruit juices.
- ➢ Helps avoid dehydration and delivers certain necessary minerals.

Full Liquid Phase

- ➢ Introduces heavier liquids and greater diversity.
- ➢ Includes protein drinks, pureed soups, and strained cream soups.
- ➢ Helps adapt the digestive system to more complex meals.

Pureed or Blended Phase

- ➢ Involves pureed or blended meals with a smooth consistency.
- ➢ Examples include infant food, yogurt, and finely pureed meats.

➢ Allows the digestive system to adapt to more solid textures.

Soft or Mechanical Soft Phase

➢ Introduces soft, easy-to-chew meals.

➢ Includes well-cooked vegetables, tender meats, and delicate fruits.

➢ Helps the person gradually return to a more normal diet.

Solid Food Phase

➢ Involves reintroducing solid meals while still concentrating on lean proteins and nutrient-dense selections.

➢ Encourages a balanced diet with a focus on protein to help muscle maintenance.

It's vital for patients who have had bariatric surgery to engage closely with a registered dietitian or healthcare professional to design a tailored plan based on their unique surgery, health state, and nutritional requirements. The dietician will generally monitor nutritional consumption, offer appropriate supplements, and give recommendations on portion management.

THE IMPORTANCE OF A BARIATRIC-FRIENDLY DIET

The Crucial Role of a Bariatric-Friendly Diet: You're Key to Success

Following bariatric surgery, or weight-loss surgery, is a big and daring step towards a healthy you. But the trip doesn't stop there. A vital, and sometimes underrated, ingredient for long-term success is adopting a bariatric-friendly diet. It's not just about calorie restriction; it's about rewiring your connection with food and optimizing the efficiency of your operation.

Promotes weight loss and maintenance

✓ **Smaller Portions, Bigger Impact**: Your bariatric operation has physically restricted your stomach size. A bariatric-friendly diet emphasizes nutrient-dense meals with fewer quantities, helping you achieve sustainable weight reduction and avoid return.

✓ **Nutrient Prioritization**: With limited space, picking the proper meals becomes crucial. This diet directs you towards protein-rich, low-fat, and low-sugar alternatives, helping you feel full while gaining critical nutrients for maximum health.

✓ **Improves Your Health**: Combating Co-morbidities Many people have bariatric surgery to treat weight-related health issues. This diet addresses those problems head-on. By lowering blood sugar, managing cholesterol, and regulating hormones, it may considerably improve illnesses including diabetes, heart disease, and sleep apnea.

✓ **Overall Wellbeing**: Beyond particular ailments, this diet supports overall well-being. Reduced inflammation, greater energy levels, and enhanced nutritional absorption all lead to a healthier, happier you.

✓ **Supports post-surgical healing and recovery**: Gentle on Your New System: The earliest phases following surgery necessitate a cautious approach. This diet delivers readily digested, liquid, and pureed meals, enabling your digestive system to repair and adapt gradually.

✓ **Nutritional Deficiencies Prevention**: Bariatric surgery affects absorption routes. This diet ensures you acquire appropriate vitamins, minerals, and electrolytes, avoiding deficiencies that might impede recovery and long-term health.

Fosters sustainable habits:

✓ **Shifting Mindsets**: This diet is not simply a temporary remedy; it's the basis for a new, better lifestyle. You'll learn to emphasize balanced meals, mindful eating, and portion control, setting you up for lasting weight management behaviors.

✓ **Empowering Choices**: With clear instructions and tasty recipes, this diet enables you to make educated food choices, promoting a feeling of control and confidence in your path.

In conclusion, a bariatric-friendly diet is not simply an afterthought; it's the cornerstone of your post-surgical success. It encourages weight reduction, improves health, supports recovery, and enables you to construct a sustainable, healthier future. Embrace it, embrace change, and embrace the life-changing opportunities that await!

TIPS FOR SUCCESS IN THE KITCHEN

The kitchen may be a battlefield or a refuge, depending on your talent and mentality. But worry not, culinary warriors! With a few simple ideas and tactics, you can convert your kitchen into a paradise of tasty successes and stress-free feasts. So, grab your whisk and sharpen your spatula, because we're about to go on a culinary journey!

Master the Mise en Place: Before the heat goes on, prep is crucial! Mise en place, a fancy French word that means "putting everything in its place," is your secret weapon for orderly cooking. Chop your vegetables, measure your seasonings, and arrange your components like a seasoned expert. This way, you can concentrate on the enjoyable part (cooking!) without searching for that elusive garlic clove.

Befriend Your Tools: A competent chef is only as good as their equipment. Invest in excellent blades that keep sharp, durable pots and pans that distribute heat uniformly, and helpful kitchen gadgets that make life simpler (hi, spiralizer!). Knowing how to utilize your equipment efficiently can raise your confidence and enhance your culinary game.

Embrace the Clean-as-You-Go Mentality: Dirty dishes stacking up may dampen even the most ardent cook's zeal. To prevent kitchen mess, use the clean-as-you-go strategy. Rinse used tools, clean up spills, and put away items as you go. This not only reduces post-meal cleaning but also keeps your desk orderly and sanitary.

Don't Fear the Flavor Fiesta: Spices are the hidden heroes of the kitchen, bringing depth, complexity, and personality to your recipes. Experiment with various spice combinations, fresh herbs, and infused oils to develop your taste characteristics. A sprinkle of za'atar, a bit of cayenne, or a spray of chile oil may transform an average meal into a tastebud journey.

Befriend Leftovers: Leftovers are not culinary failures; they're possibilities for creative reinvention! Leftover chicken may become a stir-fry filling, roasted vegetables can transform into a robust soup, and leftover rice can be the basis for wonderful fried rice. Get creative and enjoy the wonder of repurposing leftovers into new and intriguing recipes.

Celebrate the Imperfections: Not every meal will be a Michelin-starred masterpiece, and that's good! Cooking is a voyage of learning and exploration. Embrace the odd burned toast or misshapen cake as stepping stones in your culinary career. The most crucial component is to have fun and enjoy the process!

Savor the Journey: Cooking is not only about satisfying bellies; it's about nurturing spirits. Slow down, absorb the fragrances, relish the textures, and share the delight of a home-cooked dinner with loved ones. Remember, the kitchen is a place for connection, creativity, and self-expression. So, grab your apron, release your inner chef, and conquer the kitchen with these techniques in hand!

GUIDELINES FOR BARIATRIC EATING

Bariatric eating entails adopting certain standards and routines to help weight reduction, facilitate healing following surgery, and provide sufficient nutrition. These parameters may change based on the kind of bariatric surgery a person has done (e.g., gastric bypass, gastric sleeve, or laparoscopic banding). Always follow the advice made by your healthcare team, as they will adjust the guidelines to your unique requirements. Here are some basic rules for bariatric eating:

GENERAL PRINCIPLES:

Follow Stages of the Bariatric Diet
➤ Progress through the clear liquid, full liquid, pureed, soft, and solid meal stages as prescribed by your healthcare team.

Small, Frequent Meals
➤ Eat small, nutrient-dense meals throughout the day.
➤ Aim for three to six small meals or snacks to reduce overeating and help digestion.

Chew Thoroughly:

➢ Chew food thoroughly to help digestion and avoid pain.

➢ Take time to appreciate and enjoy your food.

Stay Hydrated

➢ Drink lots of water throughout the day to avoid dehydration.

➢ Avoid drinking with meals to avoid overstretching the stomach pouch.

Avoid High-Calorie, Low-Nutrient Foods

➢ Choose nutrient-dense foods such as lean protein, fruits, vegetables, and whole grains.

➢ Limit or avoid high-calorie, low-nutrient items such as sugary snacks and drinks.

NUTRIENT FOCUS

Prioritize Protein

➢ Consume protein-rich diets to enhance muscle maintenance and improve satiety.

➢ Include sources include lean meats, poultry, fish, eggs, dairy, and plant-based proteins.

Limit carbs

➢ Choose complex carbs such as whole grains, fruits, and vegetables.

➢ Limit simple sugars and processed carbs.

Monitor Fat Intake

➢ Choose healthy fats from sources including avocados, nuts, seeds, and olive oil.

➢ Limit saturated and Trans fats.

NUTRITIONAL SUPPLEMENTS

Take Recommended Supplements

➢ Follow your healthcare team's recommendations for vitamin and mineral supplements.

➢ Common supplements may include multivitamins, calcium, vitamin D, and B vitamins.

LIFESTYLE HABITS

Mindful Eating

➢ Pay attention to hunger and fullness signs.

➢ Avoid distractions when eating, such as watching TV or using technological gadgets.

Frequent Physical exercise

➢ Engage in frequent, moderate physical exercise as suggested by your healthcare team.

➢ Exercise aids weight reduction, increases mood, and enhances general well-being.

Frequent Follow-Up

➢ Attend frequent follow-up consultations with your healthcare team.

➢ Discuss any problems or difficulties connected to your nutrition and general health.

PORTION CONTROL

Portion control is a critical element of keeping a healthy diet, and it becomes more essential for persons who have had bariatric surgery or are working on weight management. Here are some recommendations for efficient portion control:

Use Smaller Plates and Bowls

➢ Opt for smaller dishware to visually fool your brain into believing you're ingesting a greater piece.

Measure and Weigh meal

➢ Use measuring cups, a kitchen scale, or visual clues to divide your meal precisely.- This helps you become more aware of optimum serving sizes.

Follow the Plate Method

➢ Divide your plate into pieces for various dietary groups: half for vegetables, one-quarter for lean protein, and one-quarter for carbs.

➢ This strategy supports a balanced and portion-controlled dinner.

Listen to Your Body

➢ Pay attention to hunger and fullness indicators.

➢ Eat carefully and quit when you feel content, not too full.

Pre Portion food

➢ Instead of eating straight from a bigger box, pre-portion food into smaller containers or baggies.

➢ This eliminates mindless snacking and helps limit calorie intake.

Avoid Second Helpings

➤ Wait a few minutes before determining whether you need seconds.

➤ Focus on tasting your food, and you may discover you're content with the original piece.

Choose Nutrient-Dense Foods

➤ Prioritize foods that are rich in nutrients, such as fruits, vegetables, lean meats, and whole grains.

➤ These meals frequently allow for greater amounts without additional calories.

Be Mindful of Liquid Calories

➤ Watch portion sizes for drinks, since liquid calories may pile up rapidly.

➤ Choose water, herbal tea, or other low-calorie choices.

Avoid Buffets and All-You-may-Eat Situations

➤ These venues may make portion control tough.

➤ Opt for ordering individual portions at restaurants instead.

Plan and Prepare Meals

➤ Plan your meals and snacks.

➤ Prepare meals at home, enabling you to manage ingredients and amounts.

Use Your Hand as a Guide

➤ Your hand may serve as a fast reference for portion amounts.

➢ For example, a portion of protein is around the size of your palm, a serving of grains or starch fits in your cupped hand, and a meal of fats should be about the size of your thumb.

Learn to Estimate Portions

➢ Develop the capacity to estimate portion proportions based on visual clues.

➢ This expertise becomes important in circumstances when measuring equipment is not accessible.

By practicing portion control, you may enjoy a variety of meals while limiting your calorie consumption and supporting your health and weight management objectives.

NUTRIENT-RICH FOODS

For persons following a bariatric diet after having weight reduction surgery, it's critical to concentrate on nutrient-dense meals that give essential vitamins and minerals while supporting weight maintenance. Here are nutrient-rich foods ideal for a bariatric diet:

LEAN PROTEINS

- Chicken Breast
- Turkey
- Fish
- Eggs
- Tofu and Tempeh

DAIRY AND DAIRY ALTERNATIVES

- Greek Yogurt
- Low-Fat Cottage Cheese
- Almond or Soy Milk

VEGETABLES

- Leafy Greens
- Broccoli
- Bell Peppers
- Cauliflower

FRUITS

- Berries
- Apples
- Pears

WHOLE GRAINS

- Quinoa
- Oats
- Brown Rice

NUTS AND SEEDS

- Almonds
- Walnuts
- Chia Seeds

LEGUMES

- Lentils
- Chickpeas
- Black Beans

HYDRATION

- Water
- Herbal teas
- Coconut water

PROTEIN SUPPLEMENTS

- Protein Shakes
- Low-sugar choices.

PORTION-CONTROLLED SNACKS:

- Greek Yogurt Cups
- Nut Packs
- String Cheese

MISCELLANEOUS

- Avocado
- Ground Flaxseed

These nutrient-rich foods may help persons following a bariatric diet achieve their nutritional demands while boosting weight reduction and maintaining overall health. It's crucial to work closely with healthcare specialists, particularly a qualified dietitian, to customize dietary advice to specific needs and post-surgery requirements. Regular monitoring and modifications to the food plan may be essential for best results.

THE IMPORTANCE OF HYDRATION

Hydration is vitally essential for persons on a bariatric diet, particularly for those who have had weight reduction surgery such as gastric bypass or gastric sleeve. Here are numerous reasons why hydration is vital in the context of a bariatric diet:

Post-Surgery Healing

✓ Adequate hydration is necessary for the healing process following bariatric surgery.

✓ Proper hydration helps tissue healing, minimizes the chance of infection, and enhances overall recovery.

Preventing Dehydration

✓ After weight reduction surgery, the stomach size is lowered, and the absorption of fluids might be adjusted.

✓ Smaller stomach capacity may result in a lower fluid intake, rendering persons more prone to dehydration.

Minimizing Constipation

✓ Dehydration may lead to constipation, a typical complication following bariatric surgery.

✓ Drinking enough water helps maintain regular bowel motions and avoids constipation.

Aiding Nutrient Absorption

✓ Hydration plays a role in the absorption of nutrients, and persons with altered gut architecture may be more sensitive to hydration status.

✓ Proper hydration helps the absorption of important vitamins and minerals from the diet.

Preventing Kidney Stones

✓ Dehydration raises the likelihood of kidney stones, a problem for certain persons undergoing bariatric surgery.

✓ Sufficient fluid intake helps avoid the production of kidney stones.

Supporting Weight Loss

✓ Staying well-hydrated may help manage appetite and reduce overeating, aiding weight reduction attempts.

✓ Sometimes, sensations of thirst might be confused for hunger, leading to needless calorie intake.

Regulating Body Temperature

✓ Hydration is vital for controlling body temperature, and persons who have had bariatric surgery may be more susceptible to temperature variations.

✓ Adequate fluid intake helps the body maintain a constant internal temperature.

Preventing Electrolyte Imbalance

✓ Proper hydration helps maintain electrolyte balance in the body.

✓ Electrolytes, such as sodium, potassium, and magnesium, play crucial roles in numerous biological activities.

HYDRATION TIPS FOR BARIATRIC PATIENTS

Sip Throughout the Day:

✓ Consume fluids gently and regularly throughout the day, as opposed to huge quantities at once.

Avoid Drinking with Meals:

✓ Limit fluid consumption during meals to prevent overstretching the stomach pouch.

✓ Wait at least 30 minutes after meals before drinking liquids.

Choose Low-Calorie, Hydrating Options:

✓ Opt for water, herbal teas, and sugar-free drinks to remain hydrated without adding additional calories.

Monitor Urine Color:

✓ Aim for light yellow urine, which is a strong sign of appropriate hydration.

✓ Dark yellow urine may signify dehydration.

Set Hydration Goals:

✓ Work with a healthcare expert to set individualized hydration goals based on individual requirements.

KITCHEN ESSENTIALS FOR BARIATRIC COOKING

Setting up a well-equipped kitchen is vital for bariatric cookery, making meal preparation easier and ensuring that persons on a bariatric diet have the tools they need for success. Here's a list of kitchen requirements for bariatric cooking:

Measuring Tools:

Measuring Cups and Spoons: Accurate portion management is vital on a bariatric diet.

Kitchen Scale: Useful for measuring food weights for proper portioning.

Small Appliances:

Blender or Food Processor: Useful for creating smoothies, purees, and soups.

Nutribullet or Personal Blender: Convenient for producing individual-sized protein shakes and smoothies.

Cookware:

Non-Stick Pans: Ideal for cooking with minimum oil.

Steamer Basket: Useful for steaming veggies while conserving their nutrients.

Baking Sheets and Pans: For roasting or baking lean meats and veggies.

Cutlery:

Quality Chef's Knife: Essential for cutting and prepping food.

Paring Knife: Useful for minor jobs and precise cutting.

Meal Prep Containers:

Portion-Controlled Containers: Aid in preparing and storing pre-portioned meals.

28 |Bariatric Diet Cookbook

Freezer-Safe Containers: Ideal for batch cooking and freezing individual servings.

Kitchen Gadgets:

Vegetable Spiralizer: Create vegetable noodles for low-carb alternatives.

Micro plane Grater: Useful for grating little quantities of cheese, citrus zest, or spices.

Vegetable Peeler: Easily peel veggies for extra convenience.

Cooking Utensils:

Tongs and Spatulas: Essential for flipping and rotating food without sticking.

Silicone Cooking Utensils: Gentle on non-stick surfaces and simple to clean.

Storage Solutions:

Food Storage Containers with Lids: For keeping cooked meals and leftovers.

Mason Jars: Useful for preserving homemade sauces, dressings, or overnight oats.

Water Bottles:

Hydration Reminder Water Bottle: Helps monitor daily water consumption.

Infuser Water Bottle: Add natural tastes to water with fruits and herbs.

Cooking Basics:

Olive Oil Sprayer: Allows for regulated usage of oil during cooking.

Herbs and Spices: Build a collection for adding taste without unnecessary salt or calories.

Low-Sodium Broths and Bouillons: Ideal for adding flavor to soups and stews.

Protein Supplements:

Protein Shaker Bottle: Convenient for mixing protein shakes.

Protein Powder: Ensure you have a high-quality, bariatric-friendly protein powder.

Dining Essentials:

Small Plates and Bowls: Encourage regulated serving proportions.

Cutlery with Comfortable Grips: Especially useful for people with dexterity difficulties post-surgery.

Educational Resources:

Cookbooks or Online dishes: Explore bariatric-friendly dishes for diversity and inspiration.

Nutritional Information Guides: Help monitor macronutrients and micronutrients in meals.

Cleaning Supplies:

Dish Soap and Scrub Brushes: Keep a clean and hygienic kitchen atmosphere.

Dish Towels and Dish Cloths: Essential for drying and wiping off surfaces.

Having these kitchen necessities available may make bariatric cooking more effective and pleasurable. Additionally, meeting with a licensed dietitian or nutritionist for individualized help on meal planning and preparation may be essential.

Batch Cooking and Freezing Tips

Batch cooking and freezing meals in advance may be a game-changer, particularly for persons on a bariatric diet. It saves time, guarantees portion control, and offers a handy solution for busy days. Here are some guidelines for good batch cooking and freezing:

BATCH COOKING TIPS:

Plan Your Menu:

Decide on a menu for the week and find dishes that can be easily scaled up for bulk cooking.

Choose Freezer-Friendly Recipes:

Not all meals freeze well. Opt for recipes that preserve their texture and taste after freezing.

Invest in Quality Containers:

Use a range of freezer-safe containers, such as portion-controlled containers, zip-top freezer bags, or glass containers with tight-fitting lids.

Label Everything:

Mark each container with the name of the meal, date of preparation, and reheating instructions.
Use a permanent marker or labels that attach well to frozen surfaces.

Cook in Batches:

Use your time productively by preparing many meals at once. For example, roast numerous chicken breasts or make a huge pot of soup.

Divide and Conquer:

Portion up recipes into individual portions before freezing. This makes it easy to defrost and reheat just what you need.

Use Your Freezer Space Wisely:

Spread containers out in the freezer to enable effective freezing. Avoid stacking containers until they are thoroughly frozen.

FREEZING TIPS:

Cool items properly:

Allow hot items to cool to room temperature before storing them in the freezer.

Divide big amounts into smaller parts to speed up the chilling process.

Avoid Freezer Burn:

Minimize air exposure by using a vacuum sealer or pressing plastic wrap firmly against the surface of items.

Remove as much air as possible from zip-top freezer bags before closing.

Flash Freezing:

Lay each portioned foods on a baking sheet to freeze separately before transferring them to a container. This stops objects from staying together.

Freeze Flat:

Store goods like soups or sauces in flat, stackable bags to conserve room in the freezer.

Once frozen, you may hold them upright for easy storage.

Organize Your Freezer:

Arrange goods in the freezer with the oldest stuff in front for easier access.

Consider utilizing boxes or baskets to classify various sorts of groceries.

Thaw Properly:

Thaw frozen meals in the refrigerator overnight for safe and even thawing.

Use the defrost option on the microwave for rapid thawing if required.

Reheat Safely:

Follow suggested reheating procedures to guarantee food safety.

Use a food thermometer to confirm that the interior temperature reaches a safe level.

Keep a Freezer Inventory:

Keep track of the goods in your freezer using an inventory list. Note the name of the meal and the day it was cooked.

BREAKFAST RECIPES

Protein Smoothie Bowl

COOKING TIME: 0 MINUTES | PREP TIME: 5 MINUTES | TOTAL TIME: 5 MINUTES | SERVING SIZE: 1 BOWL

Ingredients:

- 1 scoop unflavored protein powder
- 1 cup unsweetened almond milk* ½ cup frozen berries (mixed or your favorite kind)
- ¼ cup plain Greek yogurt (non-fat or 2%)
- ¼ cup spinach
- ½ banana
- ¼ teaspoon ground cinnamon
- Toppings (optional): unsweetened chopped nuts, seeds, berries, chia seeds, or a drizzle of sugar-free syrup

Directions:

1. Add all ingredients to a blender and blend until smooth and creamy.
2. Pour the smoothie into a bowl.
3. Top with your favorite toppings, like nuts, seeds, berries, chia seeds, or a drizzle of sugar-free syrup.

Nutritional Information (per serving): Calories: 350, Protein: 30g, Carbohydrates: 35g Fiber: 8g, Fat: 5

Tips:

- If you find the smoothie bowl too thick, add a little more almond milk or water.
- For a sweeter bowl, use ripe banana or add a few drops of stevia.
- If you don't have spinach, you can use another leafy green like kale or romaine lettuce.
- Feel free to get creative with your toppings!

Egg Muffins

PREP TIME: 5 MINUTES COOK TIME: 5 MINUTES TOTAL TIME: 10 MINUTES | SERVING SIZE: 1 WAFFLE

Ingredients:

- 1/2 cup almond flour
- 1/4 cup unsweetened almond milk
- 1/4 cup unsweetened applesauce
- 1 egg
- 1/2 teaspoon baking powder
- 1/4 teaspoon cinnamon
- Pinch of salt
- Optional toppings:
- Fresh berries
- Unsweetened Greek yogurt
- Nut butter
- Sugar-free syrup

Directions:

1. In a medium bowl, whisk together the almond flour, baking powder, cinnamon, and salt.
2. In a separate bowl, whisk together the almond milk, applesauce, and egg.
3. Pour the wet ingredients into the dry ingredients and stir until just combined. Do not over mix.
4. Heat your waffle iron according to the manufacturer's instructions. Spray with cooking spray if desired.
5. Pour about 1/4 cup of batter onto the waffle iron and cook for 3-5 minutes, or until golden brown and crispy.
6. Repeat with remaining batter.
7. Serve waffles warm with your desired toppings.

Nutritional Information per Waffle: Calories: 180, Carbohydrates: 10g (net 3g), Fiber: 3g

Fat: 12g, Protein: 10g

Tips:

- For a thicker waffle, use 1/3 cup of almond milk.
- If you don't have applesauce, you can use mashed banana or pumpkin puree.
- Add a teaspoon of vanilla extract for extra flavor.
- Store leftover waffles in an airtight container in the refrigerator for up to 3 days.

Greek Yogurt Parfait

PREP TIME: 5 MINUTES | COOKING TIME: 0 MINUTES |TOTAL TIME: 5 MINUTES | SERVING SIZE: 1

Ingredients:

- 5 Oz plain, non-fat Greek yogurt
- ¼ cup unsweetened berries (such as blueberries, raspberries, or strawberries)
- 2 tablespoons unsweetened chopped nuts (such as almonds, walnuts, or pecans)
- ¼ teaspoon ground cinnamon (optional)
- Stevia or monk fruit sweetener to taste (optional)

Directions:

1. In a small bowl, stir together the Greek yogurt, berries, and cinnamon (if using).
2. Divide the yogurt mixture evenly into two small parfait glasses or bowls.
3. Sprinkle each parfait with chopped nuts.
4. Drizzle with stevia or monk fruit sweetener to taste (optional).

Nutritional Information: Calories: 200, Protein: 20g, Carbohydrates: 15g, Fat: 5g, Fiber: 2g

Tips:

- For a thicker parfait, use thicker Greek yogurt.
- You can also use frozen berries, but thaw them slightly before adding them to the yogurt.
- If you don't have nuts, you can use a sprinkle of granola or chia seeds instead.
- Be sure to check the labels of your yogurt and sweetener to ensure they are bariatric-friendly.

Quinoa Breakfast Bowl

COOKING TIME: 15 MINUTES | PREP TIME: 5 MINUTES | TOTAL TIME: 20 MINUTES | SERVING SIZE: 1 BOWL

Ingredients:

- 1/2 cup quinoa, rinsed
- 1 cup unsweetened almond milk (or any milk of your choice)
- 1/4 cup berries (mixed or your favorite kind)
- 1/4 cup chopped nuts or seeds (pumpkin, sunflower, almonds, etc.)
- 1/4 cup Greek yogurt (low-fat or fat-free)
- 1/4 teaspoon cinnamon
- 1/4 teaspoon ground ginger
- Honey or maple syrup (optional, to taste)

Directions:

1. In a saucepan, combine quinoa and almond milk. Bring to a boil, then reduce heat, cover, and simmer for 15 minutes, or until quinoa is cooked and fluffy.
2. While the quinoa is cooking, prepare your toppings. Wash and chop the berries, and toast the nuts or seeds if desired.
3. Once the quinoa is cooked, fluff it with a fork and divide it into a bowl. Top with the berries, nuts/seeds, Greek yogurt, cinnamon, and ginger. Drizzle with honey or maple syrup, if using.

Nutritional Information (per serving): Calories: 250, Protein: 15g, Carbohydrates: 35g, Fiber: 5g, Fat: 5g

Tips:

- For added protein, you can stir in a scoop of protein powder before serving.
- Feel free to get creative with your toppings! Other delicious options include chopped banana, mango, chia seeds, or a drizzle of nut butter.
- Leftovers can be stored in an airtight container in the refrigerator for up to 3 days.

Cottage Cheese and Fruit Salad

PREP TIME: 10 MINUTES | COOKING TIME: 0 MINUTES | TOTAL TIME: 10 MINUTES | SERVING SIZE: 1 CUP

Ingredients:

- 1 cup low-fat or non-fat cottage cheese
- 1/2 cup chopped fresh fruit (such as berries, melon, apple, pear)
- 1/4 cup chopped celery or cucumber (optional)
- 1 tablespoon chopped nuts or seeds (optional)
- 1 teaspoon ground cinnamon or nutmeg (optional)
- 1 tablespoon light salad dressing (optional)

Instructions:

1. In a bowl, combine the cottage cheese, fruit, celery or cucumber (if using), nuts or seeds (if using), and cinnamon or nutmeg (if using).
2. Toss gently to combine.
3. If desired, drizzle with light salad dressing just before serving.

Nutritional Information (per serving): Calories: 150, Protein: 18g, Fat: 5g, Carbohydrates: 15g, Fiber: 3g, Sugar: 5g

Tips:

- For a sweeter salad, use ripe fruits with higher natural sugar content.
- You can also add a touch of sweetness with a dash of artificial sweetener.
- If you're on a strict bariatric diet, it's best to skip the salad dressing or choose a sugar-free option.
- This salad is also a great source of calcium, which is important for bone health after bariatric surgery.

Chia Seed Pudding

COOKING TIME: 0 MINUTES (just prep and refrigerate) | PREP TIME: 5 MINUTES | TOTAL TIME: 5 MINUTES (plus overnight refrigeration) | SERVING SIZE: 1 CUP

Ingredients:

- 1/4 cup chia seeds
- 1 cup unsweetened almond milk (or other low-fat milk)
- 1/4 cup unsweetened Greek yogurt (optional)
- 1/2 teaspoon vanilla extract
- 1/4 teaspoon ground cinnamon
- Pinch of stevia or other sweetener (optional)
- Toppings (optional): fresh fruit, nuts, seeds, shredded coconut, cocoa nibs

Directions:

1. Combine chia seeds, almond milk, yogurt (if using), vanilla extract, cinnamon, and sweetener (if using) in a bowl or jar. Stir well to combine.
2. Cover the bowl or jar and refrigerate for at least 2 hours, or overnight, until the pudding has thickened.
3. When ready to serve, stir the pudding again and top with your favorite toppings.

Nutritional information (per serving): Calories: 240, Carbohydrates: 12g (5g fiber), Protein: 6g, Fat: 14g

Tips:

- For a thicker pudding, use less liquid.
- For a sweeter pudding, add more sweetener to taste.
- You can use any type of milk you like, but unsweetened almond milk or another low-fat milk is best for a bariatric diet.
- You can also add other spices to the pudding, such as nutmeg, ginger, or cardamom.
- If you don't have fresh fruit, you can use frozen fruit or canned fruit in light syrup.

Vegetable Omelet

PREP TIME: 5 MINUTES | COOK TIME: 10 MINUTES | TOTAL TIME: 15 MINUTES | SERVING SIZE: 1

Ingredients:

- 2 whole eggs
- 2 large egg whites
- 1/4 cup chopped bell pepper (any color)
- 1/4 cup chopped onion
- 1/4 cup chopped spinach
- 1/4 cup chopped mushrooms
- 1/4 cup shredded low-fat cheese (optional)
- 1 tablespoon olive oil
- Salt and pepper to taste

Directions:

1. In a small bowl, whisk together the eggs and egg whites. Season with salt and pepper.

2. Heat the olive oil in a non-stick skillet over medium heat. Add the bell pepper, onion, spinach, and mushrooms, and cook until softened, about 3-5 minutes.

3. Pour the egg mixture into the skillet and spread it evenly. Let cook for about 2-3 minutes, or until the bottom is set.

4. If desired, sprinkle the cheese over one half of the omelet. Fold the other half over the cheese to make a half-moon shape.

5. Cook for another minute or two, until the cheese is melted and the omelet is cooked through.

6. Slide the omelet onto a plate and serve immediately.

Nutritional Information (per serving): Calories: 220, Carbohydrates: 5 grams, Fiber: 3 grams, Protein: 20 grams, Fat: 10 grams

Tips:

- For a vegan option, use chickpea flour or tofu scramble instead of eggs.
- Add other vegetables to your liking, such as broccoli, zucchini, or tomatoes.
- Serve the omelet with a side of whole-wheat toast or fruit salad for a complete meal.

Ricotta and Berry Stuffed Crepes

PREP TIME: 10 MINUTES | COOK TIME: 15 MINUTES |TOTAL TIME: 25 MINUTES | SERVING SIZE: 2 CREPES

Ingredients:

For the crepes:

- 1/2 cup whole wheat flour
- 1/4 cup unsweetened almond milk
- 1/4 cup water
- 1 egg
- 1/4 teaspoon vanilla extract
- Pinch of salt

For the filling:

- 1/4 cup low-fat ricotta cheese
- 1/4 cup mixed berries (strawberries, blueberries, raspberries)
- 1 tablespoon chopped fresh mint (optional)
- 1 teaspoon honey (optional)

Directions:

1. Make the crepes: In a blender, combine the flour, almond milk, water, egg, vanilla extract, and salt. Blend until smooth.
2. Heat a lightly greased non-stick skillet over medium heat. Pour about 1/4 cup of batter into the pan, swirling to form a thin circle. Cook for 1-2 minutes per side, or until golden brown. Repeat with remaining batter.
3. Make the filling: In a small bowl, combine the ricotta cheese, berries, and mint (if using). If desired, add a touch of honey for sweetness.
4. Assemble the crepes: Spread a spoonful of the ricotta-berry mixture onto each crepe. Fold in half or roll up, and enjoy!

Nutritional information per serving (approximate): Calories: 200, Protein: 15g, Fat: 5g, Carbohydrates: 25g, Fiber: 3g, Sugar: 5g

Tips:

- For a protein boost, add a scoop of protein powder to the crepe batter.
- Use any type of berries you like. Frozen berries can be used if fresh are not available.
- If you prefer a sweeter crepe, add a sprinkle of cinnamon or nutmeg to the batter.
- Serve with a dollop of low-fat Greek yogurt or unsweetened whipped cream for added richness.

Oatmeal with Nut Butter

COOKING TIME: 5 MINUTES |PREP TIME: 5 MINUTES |TOTAL TIME: 10 MINUTES |SERVING SIZE: 1 CUP

Ingredients:

- 1/2 cup rolled oats
- 1 cup unsweetened almond milk (or other plant-based milk)
- 1/4 cup unsweetened applesauce
- 2 tablespoons natural nut butter (almond, peanut, cashew, etc.)
- 1/4 teaspoon ground cinnamon
- Pinch of salt (optional)
- Toppings (optional): fresh berries, chopped nuts, seeds, sliced banana

Directions:

1. In a saucepan, combine oats and almond milk. Bring to a boil, then reduce heat and simmer for 5 minutes, or until oats are cooked through.
2. Stir in applesauce, nut butter, cinnamon, and salt (if using).
3. Remove from heat and serve immediately.
4. Top with your favorite toppings, if desired.

Nutritional Information (per serving): Calories: 250, Protein: 15g, Fat: 10g, Carbohydrates: 30g, Fiber: 5g, Sugar: 5g

Tips:

- For a thicker oatmeal, cook for an additional minute or two.
- If you don't have applesauce, you can use mashed banana or another type of fruit puree.
- You can also add a scoop of protein powder to boost the protein content.
- Be sure to choose a natural nut butter without added sugar or unhealthy fats.
- This recipe is easily customizable to your taste. Feel free to experiment with different nut butters, spices, and toppings.

Turkey Sausage and Spinach Breakfast Casserole

COOKING TIME: 25-30 MINUTES | PREP TIME: 10 MINUTES | TOTAL TIME: 35-40 MINUTES | SERVING SIZE: 1/6 OF THE CASSEROLE

Ingredients:

- 1/2 pound lean ground turkey sausage (90% lean or higher)
- 1 tablespoon olive oil
- 1/2 onion, chopped
- 2 cloves garlic, minced
- 10 Oz fresh spinach, chopped
- 1/2 cup chopped bell pepper (any color)
- 1 cup chopped mushrooms (optional)
- 1/2 cup fat-free Greek yogurt
- 1/4 cup low-fat milk
- 2 large eggs, whisked
- 1/4 cup reduced-fat shredded cheddar cheese
- 1/4 teaspoon dried thyme
- 1/4 teaspoon dried oregano
- Salt and pepper to taste

Directions:

1. Preheat oven to 375°F (190°C). Grease an 8x8 inch baking dish.
2. In a large skillet over medium heat, brown the turkey sausage with olive oil. Drain excess fat.
3. Add onion and garlic to the skillet and cook until softened, about 3-5 minutes.
4. Stir in spinach, bell pepper, and mushrooms (if using) and cook until spinach is wilted, about 2-3 minutes.
5. In a bowl, whisk together Greek yogurt, milk, eggs, cheese, thyme, oregano, salt, and pepper.
6. Pour the yogurt mixture into the skillet with the sausage and vegetables. Stir to combine.
7. Transfer the mixture to the prepared baking dish.
8. Bake for 25-30 minutes, or until the casserole is set and bubbly.
9. Let cool slightly before serving.

Nutritional Information (per serving): Calories: 180, Protein: 20g, Fat: 6g, Carbohydrates: 12g, Fiber: 4g

Sweet Potato Hash

PREP TIME: 10 MINUTES | COOK TIME: 20 MINUTES | TOTAL TIME: 30 MINUTES | SERVING SIZE: 1 CUP

Ingredients:

- 1 medium sweet potato, peeled and diced
- 1/2 bell pepper, any color, diced
- 1/4 onion, diced
- 2 cloves garlic, minced
- 1/4 cup cooked lean protein (chicken, turkey, tofu, etc.)
- 1/4 cup low-fat Greek yogurt or cottage cheese
- 1 tablespoon olive oil
- 1/2 teaspoon dried herbs (such as rosemary, thyme, or oregano)
- Salt and pepper to taste

Directions:

1. Preheat oven to 400°F (200°C).
2. Toss diced sweet potato, bell pepper, onion, and garlic with olive oil and herbs in a large bowl. Season with salt and pepper.
3. Spread the mixture evenly on a baking sheet.
4. Bake for 20 minutes, or until the sweet potatoes are tender and slightly browned.
5. While the hash is baking, cook your protein of choice according to package instructions.
6. Once the hash is cooked, stir in the cooked protein and yogurt or cottage cheese.
7. Serve immediately and enjoy!

Nutritional Information (per serving): Calories: 250, Carbohydrates: 35g, Protein: 15g, Fat: 5g, Fiber: 5g

Tips:

- For a spicier hash, add a pinch of cayenne pepper or chili flakes.
- You can add other vegetables to the hash, such as zucchini, mushrooms, or spinach.
- Leftovers can be stored in an airtight container in the refrigerator for up to 3 days.

Peanut Butter Banana Wrap

COOKING TIME: N/A | PREP TIME: 5 MINUTES | TOTAL TIME: 5 MINUTES | SERVING SIZE: 1 WRAP

Ingredients:

- 1 whole-wheat tortilla (60-70 calories)
- 2 tablespoons natural peanut butter (190 calories)
- 1 ripe banana, sliced
- ¼ cup chopped almonds (60 calories)
- ¼ teaspoon cinnamon (optional)

Directions:

1. Spread the peanut butter evenly on the tortilla.
2. Top with the banana slices and sprinkle with almonds and cinnamon (if using).
3. Roll up the tortilla tightly and enjoy!

Nutritional Information (per serving): Calories: 250, Protein: 15g, Fat: 8g, Carbohydrates: 30g, Fiber: 4g, Sugar: 10g

Tips:

- For a vegan option, use natural almond butter or another type of nut butter.
- You can add other toppings to your liking, such as berries, sliced apples, or shredded coconut.
- If you're not a fan of peanut butter, you can use mashed avocado instead.
- This wrap is best enjoyed fresh, but you can store it in the refrigerator for up to 24 hours.

Smoked Salmon and Cream Cheese Roll-Ups

COOKING TIME: N/A (NO COOKING REQUIRED) | PREP TIME: 10 MINUTES | TOTAL TIME: 10 MINUTES | SERVING SIZE: 10 ROLL-UPS (ADJUST AS NEEDED)

Ingredients:

- 4 large romaine lettuce leaves
- 4 oz. light cream cheese (whipped or spreadable)
- 4 oz. thin-sliced smoked salmon
- 1/4 cup chopped chives (optional)
- Freshly ground black pepper, to taste

Directions:

1. Wash and dry the romaine lettuce leaves.
2. Spread a thin layer of cream cheese onto each lettuce leaf.
3. Top with smoked salmon slices.
4. Sprinkle with chives and black pepper, if desired.
5. Roll up the lettuce leaves tightly, like cigarillos.
6. Cut each roll-up into bite-sized pieces and enjoy!

Nutritional information per serving: Calories: 120, Protein: 8g, Fat: 7g, Carbohydrates: 2g

Tips:

- For a vegan option, use a dairy-free cream cheese alternative.
- You can add other fillings to your roll-ups, such as cucumber slices, dill, or red onion.
- If you prefer a warmer snack, briefly toast the lettuce leaves in a dry pan before spreading with cream cheese.
- Store leftover roll-ups in an airtight container in the refrigerator for up to 2 days.

Protein Pancakes

PREP TIME: 5 MINUTES | COOKING TIME: 10 MINUTES | TOTAL TIME: 15 MINUTES | SERVING SIZE: 1 PANCAKE

Ingredients

- 1/4 cup plain Greek yogurt
- 1/4 cup unsweetened almond milk
- 1/4 cup rolled oats
- 1 scoop vanilla protein powder
- 1/2 teaspoon baking powder
- 1/4 teaspoon cinnamon (optional)
- Pinch of salt

Directions:

1. In a blender or food processor, combine all ingredients until smooth.
2. Heat a lightly greased skillet or griddle over medium heat.
3. Pour about 1/4 cup of batter per pancake onto the skillet.
4. Cook for 2-3 minutes per side, or until golden brown and cooked through.
5. Serve immediately with your favorite bariatric-friendly toppings.

Nutritional Information (per pancake): Calories: 150, Protein: 18g, Carbohydrates: 15g, Fiber: 3g, Fat: 3g

Tips:

- For extra protein, add a chopped hard-boiled egg or a tablespoon of chia seeds to the batter.
- Get creative with toppings! Try fresh berries, a dollop of Greek yogurt, or a sprinkle of nuts or seeds.
- These pancakes can be stored in an airtight container in the refrigerator for up to 3 days. Reheat in a microwave or oven until warmed through.

Avocado and Tomato Toast

PREP TIME: 10 MINUTES | COOKING TIME: NONE | TOTAL TIME: 10 MINUTES | SERVING SIZE: 1 SLICE OF TOAST

Ingredients:

- 1 slice whole-wheat or protein bread
- 1/4 ripe avocado, mashed
- 1/2 medium tomato, sliced
- 1/4 cup baby spinach
- 1 tablespoon crumbled goat cheese (optional)
- Pinch of salt and pepper
- Squeeze of lemon juice (optional)

Directions:

1. Toast the bread until golden brown.
2. While the bread is toasting, mash the avocado with a fork until smooth.
3. Spread the mashed avocado onto the toast.
4. Top with the sliced tomato and baby spinach.
5. Season with salt and pepper, and a squeeze of lemon juice if desired.
6. Optionally, add crumbled goat cheese for a bit of creaminess and protein.

Nutritional Information (per serving): Calories: 240, Carbohydrates: 28g (net 18g), Fat: 14g (monounsaturated), Fiber: 8g, Protein: 4g, Vitamin C: 30% DV, Potassium: 15% DV, Vitamin K: 10% DV

Tips:

- To ripen an avocado quickly, place it in a brown paper bag with a banana or apple.
- Add other bariatric-friendly toppings like sliced cucumber, red onion, or sprouts.
- Use a protein bread for an extra boost of protein.
- For a richer flavor, drizzle the toast with balsamic vinegar or a light olive oil.

Shrimp and Veggie Stir-Fry

COOKING TIME: 10 MINUTES | PREP TIME: 10 MINUTES | TOTAL TIME: 20 MINUTES | SERVING SIZE: 1 CUP

Ingredients:

- 4 ounces raw shrimp, peeled and deveined
- 1 tablespoon olive oil
- 1/2 cup broccoli florets
- 1/2 cup red bell pepper, sliced
- 1/2 cup green bell pepper, sliced
- 1/4 cup sugar snap peas
- 1 clove garlic, minced
- 1/4 cup low-sodium chicken broth
- 1 tablespoon low-sodium soy sauce
- 1/2 teaspoon cornstarch
- 1/4 teaspoon black pepper
- 1/4 teaspoon red pepper flakes (optional)
- 1 tablespoon chopped fresh cilantro

Directions:

1. Prep the shrimp: Pat the shrimp dry with paper towels. If desired, you can cut them into smaller pieces.
2. Heat the oil: In a large skillet or wok over medium-high heat, heat the olive oil.
3. Cook the shrimp: Add the shrimp to the pan and cook for 2-3 minutes per side, or until pink and cooked through. Remove from the pan and set aside.
4. Sauté the veggies: Add the broccoli, red bell pepper, green bell pepper, and sugar snap peas to the pan. Cook for 3-4 minutes, or until crisp-tender.
5. Add the garlic: Add the garlic to the pan and cook for 30 seconds, until fragrant.
6. Make the sauce: In a small bowl, whisk together the chicken broth, soy sauce, cornstarch, black pepper, and red pepper flakes (if using).
7. Thicken the sauce: Add the sauce to the pan and bring to a simmer. Cook for 1 minute, or until slightly thickened.
8. Return the shrimp: Add the cooked shrimp back to the pan and toss to combine.
9. Garnish and serve: Garnish with chopped cilantro and serve immediately.

Nutritional Information (per serving): Calories: 250, Protein: 25 grams, Carbohydrates: 15 grams, Fiber: 3 grams, Fat: 5 grams

Spinach and Feta Egg Wrap

COOKING TIME: 5 MINUTES | PREP TIME: 5 MINUTES | TOTAL TIME: 10 MINUTES | SERVING SIZE: 1 WRAP

Ingredients:

- 1 whole egg
- 2 large egg whites
- 1/4 cup chopped spinach
- 1/4 ounce crumbled feta cheese
- 1/4 teaspoon chopped fresh dill (optional)
- Salt and pepper to taste
- 1 whole wheat tortilla

Directions:

1. In a small bowl, whisk together the whole egg and egg whites.
2. Heat a nonstick skillet over medium heat. Spray with cooking spray if desired.
3. Pour the egg mixture into the skillet and spread into a thin omelet.
4. Cook for 2-3 minutes, or until the eggs are just set.
5. Sprinkle the spinach over the eggs and cook for another minute, or until wilted.
6. Remove the skillet from the heat and let the eggs cool slightly.
7. Spread the feta cheese and dill (if using) over the eggs.
8. Season with salt and pepper to taste.
9. Place the tortilla on a flat surface. Place the egg mixture in the center of the tortilla.
10. Fold the bottom of the tortilla up over the eggs, then fold in the sides. Roll up the tortilla tightly.
11. Cut the wrap in half and enjoy!

Nutritional information per serving (approximate): Calories: 250, Protein: 20g, Carbs: 10g, Fat: 15g

Mango Coconut Chia Pudding

COOKING TIME: NONE | PREP TIME: 10 MINUTES | TOTAL TIME: 10 MINUTES (PLUS OVERNIGHT CHILLING) | SERVING SIZE: 1 CUP (240 ML)

Nutritional Information (per serving): Calories: 240, Fat: 13 grams (saturated 8 grams), Carbohydrates: 22 grams (fiber 9 grams, sugar 13 grams), Protein: 5 grams

Ingredients:

- 1/2 cup unsweetened plain almond milk (or other unsweetened milk)
- 1/4 cup unsweetened light coconut milk
- 2 tablespoons chia seeds
- 1/2 teaspoon vanilla extract
- 1/4 teaspoon ground cinnamon
- Pinch of salt
- 1/2 cup fresh mango, diced
- 1 tablespoon unsweetened shredded coconut (optional)

Directions:

1. In a small bowl or jar, whisk together the almond milk, coconut milk, chia seeds, vanilla extract, cinnamon, and salt. Let sit for 5 minutes, or until the chia seeds begin to thicken.
2. Stir in the diced mango. Cover and refrigerate for at least 4 hours, or overnight, for best results.
3. When ready to serve, stir the pudding again and top with unsweetened shredded coconut, if desired.

Tips:

For a thicker pudding, use a ratio of 3 tablespoons chia seeds to 1/2 cup liquid.

You can use any type of milk you like, but unsweetened almond milk or coconut milk are good choices for a bariatric diet.

If you don't have fresh mango, you can use frozen mango that has been thawed.

You can add other toppings to your liking, such as berries, nuts, or seeds.

Caprese Breakfast Skewers

COOKING TIME: 5 MINUTES | PREP TIME: 10 MINUTES | TOTAL TIME: 15 MINUTES | SERVING SIZE: 1 SKEWER

Ingredients:

- 4 cherry tomatoes
- 4 bocconcini mozzarella balls
- 4 fresh basil leaves
- 1 tablespoon olive oil
- 1/4 teaspoon dried oregano
- Pinch of salt and pepper
- 4 bamboo skewers

Directions:

1. Wash the cherry tomatoes and basil leaves.
2. cut the tomatoes in half and the mozzarella balls into bite-sized pieces.
3. In a small bowl, whisk together the olive oil, oregano, salt, and pepper.
4. Thread the tomatoes, mozzarella balls, and basil leaves onto the skewers, alternating the ingredients.
5. Drizzle the skewers with the dressing.
6. Serve immediately.

Nutritional information (per skewer): Calories: 150, Protein: 10g, Fat: 8g, Carbs: 5g, Fiber: 2g

Tips:

- For a vegan option, use cherry tomatoes, marinated tofu cubes, and fresh basil leaves.
- If you don't have bamboo skewers, you can use toothpicks.
- You can also make these skewers ahead of time and store them in the refrigerator for up to 24 hours.

Almond Flour Waffles

PREP TIME: 5 MINUTES | COOK TIME: 5 MINUTES | TOTAL TIME: 10 MINUTES | SERVING SIZE: 1 WAFFLE

Ingredients:

- 1/2 cup almond flour
- 1/4 cup unsweetened almond milk
- 1/4 cup unsweetened applesauce
- 1 egg
- 1/2 teaspoon baking powder
- 1/4 teaspoon cinnamon
- Pinch of salt
- **Optional toppings:**
- Fresh berries
- Unsweetened Greek yogurt
- Nut butter
- Sugar-free syrup

Instructions:

1. In a medium bowl, whisk together the almond flour, baking powder, cinnamon, and salt.
2. In a separate bowl, whisk together the almond milk, applesauce, and egg.
3. Pour the wet ingredients into the dry ingredients and stir until just combined. Do not over mix.
4. Heat your waffle iron according to the manufacturer's instructions. Spray with cooking spray if desired.
5. Pour about 1/4 cup of batter onto the waffle iron and cook for 3-5 minutes, or until golden brown and crispy.
6. Repeat with remaining batter.
7. Serve waffles warm with your desired toppings.

Nutritional Information per Waffle: Calories: 180, Carbohydrates: 10g (net 3g), Fiber: 3g, Fat: 12g, Protein: 10g

LUNCH RECIPES

Grilled Chicken Salad

COOKING TIME: 10 MINUTES (grilling chicken) | PREP TIME: 10 MINUTES | TOTAL TIME: 20 MINUTES | SERVING SIZE: 1 LARGE SALAD (approximately 2 cups)

Ingredients:

- 4 Oz boneless, skinless chicken breast
- 1 cup mixed greens (spinach, romaine, kale)
- 1/2 cup chopped cucumber
- 1/2 cup chopped tomato
- 1/4 cup diced red onion
- 1/4 cup crumbled feta cheese
- 2 tablespoons light balsamic vinaigrette dressing
- Salt and pepper to taste
- Optional: Herbs like basil, oregano, or parsley for garnish

Directions:

1. Prepare the chicken: Preheat a grill pan or grill to medium-high heat. Season the chicken breast with salt and pepper to taste.
2. Grill the chicken: Grill the chicken breast for 5-7 minutes per side, or until cooked through. Let cool slightly and then slice or chop into bite-sized pieces.
3. Assemble the salad: In a large bowl, combine the mixed greens, cucumber, tomato, red onion, and feta cheese.
4. Add the protein: Top the salad with the grilled chicken pieces.
5. Dress and season: Drizzle the salad with the balsamic vinaigrette dressing, and season with additional salt and pepper to taste. Garnish with fresh herbs if desired.

Nutritional Information (per serving): Calories: 350, Protein: 35g, Carbohydrates: 15g (including 5g fiber), Fat: 5g

Tuna Lettuce Wraps

COOKING TIME: N/A | PREP TIME: 10 MINUTES | TOTAL TIME: 10 MINUTES | SERVING SIZE: 4 WRAPS

Ingredients:

- 4 large romaine lettuce leaves
- 6 Oz canned tuna packed in water, drained and flaked
- 1/4 cup chopped celery
- 1/4 cup chopped red onion
- 1 tablespoon light mayonnaise (or Greek yogurt for a lower-fat option)
- 1 tablespoon Dijon mustard
- 1 tablespoon lemon juice
- 1/4 teaspoon dried dill
- Salt and pepper to taste
- Optional toppings: chopped tomato, cucumber, avocado, sprouts, cilantro

Directions:

1. Wash and dry the romaine lettuce leaves.
2. In a medium bowl, combine the tuna, celery, red onion, mayonnaise (or Greek yogurt), Dijon mustard, lemon juice, dill, salt, and pepper. Mix well.
3. Fill each lettuce leaf with about 1/4 cup of the tuna mixture.
4. Top with your desired toppings and enjoy!

Nutritional Information (per wrap): Calories: 150, Carbohydrates: 4g, Fat: 5g, Protein: 20g

Tips:

- For a spicier wrap, add a pinch of red pepper flakes to the tuna mixture.
- If you're short on time, you can use pre-chopped celery and red onion.
- To make this recipe ahead of time, assemble the wraps and store them in the refrigerator for up to 24 hours.
- Feel free to get creative with your toppings! Other delicious options include shredded carrots, bell peppers, or crumbled feta cheese.

Zucchini Noodles with Pesto and Cherry Tomatoes

COOKING TIME: 10 MINUTES | PREP TIME: 10 MINUTES | TOTAL TIME: 20 MINUTES | SERVING SIZE: 1 CUP

Ingredients:

- 2 medium zucchinis
- 1/3 cup store-bought pesto (or homemade, if preferred)
- 1/2 cup cherry tomatoes, halved
- 1 tablespoon olive oil
- 1/4 cup crumbled feta cheese (optional)
- Freshly ground black pepper, to taste

Directions:

1. Wash and dry the zucchinis. Using a spiralizer, create long, thin noodles from the zucchinis.
2. Heat the olive oil in a large skillet over medium heat. Add the zucchini noodles and cook for 5-7 minutes, until tender-crisp.
3. Stir in the pesto and cherry tomatoes, and cook for an additional 2-3 minutes, until warmed through.
4. Remove from heat and season with black pepper to taste.
5. Serve immediately, topped with crumbled feta cheese (optional).

Nutritional Information (per serving): Calories: 250, Protein: 10g, Fat: 15g, Carbohydrates: 15g, Fiber: 5g

Tips:

- For a richer flavor, add a drizzle of balsamic glaze or a squeeze of fresh lemon juice before serving.
- If you don't have a spiralizer, you can use a julienne peeler to create thin zucchini strips.
- You can also add other vegetables to this dish, such as roasted bell peppers, chopped spinach, or shredded carrots.
- This dish can be stored in an airtight container in the refrigerator for up to 2 days.

Quinoa and Black Bean Bowl

COOKING TIME: 20 MINUTES | PREP TIME: 10 MINUTES | TOTAL TIME: 30 MINUTES | SERVING SIZE: 1 BOWL

Ingredients:

- 1 cup quinoa, rinsed
- 1 1/2 cups vegetable broth
- 1 can (15 Oz) black beans, rinsed and drained
- 1/2 cup chopped red bell pepper
- 1/4 cup chopped red onion
- 1/4 cup chopped cilantro
- 1 tablespoon olive oil
- 1 tablespoon lime juice
- 1/2 teaspoon chili powder
- 1/4 teaspoon cumin
- Salt and pepper to taste

- **Optional toppings:**
- Avocado slices
- Salsa
- Chopped fresh mango
- Greek yogurt
- Hot sauce

Directions:

1. In a saucepan, combine quinoa and vegetable broth. Bring to a boil, then reduce heat to low, cover, and simmer for 20 minutes, or until all liquid is absorbed.
2. While quinoa is cooking, heat olive oil in a skillet over medium heat. Add bell pepper and onion, and cook for 5-7 minutes, until softened.
3. Stir in black beans, chili powder, cumin, salt, and pepper. Cook for an additional 3-4 minutes, until heated through.
4. Fluff cooked quinoa with a fork.
5. Divide quinoa evenly into bowls. Top with black beans, cilantro, and your desired toppings. Drizzle with lime juice before serving.

Nutritional Information (per serving): Calories: 300, Protein: 15g, Carbohydrates: 45g, Fiber: 8g, Fat: 5g

Salmon and Avocado Sushi Bowl

COOKING TIME: 15 MINUTES | PREP TIME: 10 MINUTES | TOTAL TIME: 25 MINUTES | SERVING SIZE: 1 BOWL

Ingredients:

- 1 cup cooked sushi rice (brown or white)
- 4 Oz salmon fillet, cooked and flaked
- 1/2 avocado, thinly sliced
- 1/2 cup cucumber, thinly sliced
- 1/4 cup carrot, julienned
- 1/4 cup edamame, shelled
- 1 tablespoon seaweed salad (optional)
- 1 tablespoon rice vinegar
- 1/2 teaspoon sesame oil
- 1/4 teaspoon wasabi paste (optional)
- Chopped fresh chives, for garnish
- Pickled ginger, for serving (optional)

Directions:

1. Cook the rice: According to package instructions, cook the sushi rice. While the rice is warm, drizzle with rice vinegar and sesame oil, and fluff gently with a fork.
2. Prepare the salmon: Cook the salmon fillet using your preferred method (baking, grilling, poaching, etc.). Flake the cooked salmon into bite-sized pieces.
3. Assemble the bowl: Divide the cooked rice evenly between two bowls. Top with the flaked salmon, avocado slices, cucumber, carrot, and edamame.
4. Add the finishing touches: If using, spoon a dollop of seaweed salad onto each bowl. Garnish with chopped chives and serve with pickled ginger and wasabi paste (optional).

Nutritional Information (per serving): Calories: 350, Protein: 30g, Carbohydrates: 35g, Fat: 15g, Fiber: 5g

Egg Salad Stuffed Bell Peppers

COOKING TIME: 10 MINUTES | PREP TIME: 15 MINUTES | TOTAL TIME: 25 MINUTES | SERVING SIZE: 1 STUFFED BELL PEPPER HALF

Ingredients:

- 1 bell pepper, any color (halved and seeded)
- 2 hard-boiled eggs, chopped
- 2 tablespoons plain Greek yogurt
- 1 tablespoon light mayonnaise
- 1/4 cup chopped celery
- 1/4 cup chopped red onion
- 1 tablespoon fresh dill, chopped (optional)
- Salt and pepper to taste

Directions:

1. Preheat oven to 375°F (190°C).
2. Place the bell pepper halves on a baking sheet, cut side down. Drizzle with a little olive oil or spray with cooking spray. Bake for 10 minutes, or until softened slightly.
3. While the peppers are baking, in a medium bowl, combine the chopped eggs, Greek yogurt, mayonnaise, celery, red onion, and dill (if using). Season with salt and pepper to taste.
4. Once the peppers are cooked, remove them from the oven and let them cool for a few minutes. Fill each half with the egg salad mixture.
5. Serve immediately or store in an airtight container in the refrigerator for up to 3 days.

Nutritional Information (per serving): Calories: 150, Protein: 12 grams, Carbohydrates: 8 grams, Fat: 5 grams, Fiber: 2 grams

Tips:

- For a creamier egg salad, add a little more Greek yogurt or mayonnaise.
- If you don't have fresh dill, you can use 1/2 teaspoon of dried dill weed.
- Feel free to add other chopped vegetables to the egg salad, such as cucumber or bell peppers.
- To make this recipe vegan, use vegan mayonnaise and tofu scramble instead of eggs.

Cauliflower Fried Rice with Shrimp

COOKING TIME: 15 MINUTES | PREP TIME: 10 MINUTES | TOTAL TIME: 25 MINUTES | SERVING SIZE: 1 CUP

Ingredients:

- 1 tablespoon avocado oil
- 1/2 small onion, diced
- 1 clove garlic, minced
- 3 cups cauliflower florets, riced (see notes)
- 1/2 pound shrimp, peeled and deveined
- 1/2 cup frozen peas
- 2 large eggs, beaten
- 2 tablespoons low-sodium soy sauce
- 1 tablespoon rice vinegar
- 1/2 teaspoon sesame oil
- 1/4 teaspoon ground ginger
- Pinch of red pepper flakes (optional)
- Green onions, sliced (for garnish)

Directions:

1. Heat avocado oil in a large skillet or wok over medium heat. Add onion and cook until softened, about 5 minutes.
2. Add garlic and cook for 30 seconds until fragrant.
3. Stir in rice cauliflower and cook for 5-7 minutes, until softened but still slightly crisp.
4. Push the cauliflower to one side of the pan and add the shrimp. Cook for 2-3 minutes per side, until pink and cooked through.
5. Add the peas and cook for another minute.
6. Push the ingredients to one side of the pan again and pour in the beaten eggs. Scramble the eggs until cooked through.
7. Stir in soy sauce, rice vinegar, sesame oil, ginger, and red pepper flakes (if using).
8. Combine everything together and cook for another minute.
9. Garnish with sliced green onions and serve immediately.

Nutritional Information per Serving: Calories: 250, Protein: 25g, Carbs: 10g (net), Fat: 8g

Caprese Chicken Skewers

COOKING TIME: 10-15 MINUTES | PREP TIME: 10 MINUTES | TOTAL TIME: 20-25 MINUTES | SERVING SIZE: 2 SKEWERS

Ingredients:

- 4 oz. boneless, skinless chicken breast, cut into bite-sized pieces
- 12 cherry tomatoes
- 4 small mozzarella balls, halved
- 12 fresh basil leaves
- 1 tablespoon olive oil
- 1/2 teaspoon dried oregano
- 1/4 teaspoon garlic powder
- Salt and pepper to taste

Directions:

1. Preheat grill or grill pan to medium-high heat.
2. In a bowl, toss chicken with olive oil, oregano, garlic powder, salt, and pepper.
3. Thread chicken, tomatoes, mozzarella, and basil leaves onto skewers, alternating ingredients.
4. Grill skewers for 10-15 minutes, or until chicken is cooked through and tomatoes are slightly softened.
5. Serve immediately with a drizzle of balsamic vinegar or a dollop of pesto (optional).

Nutritional Information (per serving): Calories: 250-300, Protein: 30-35g, Fat: 10-15g, Carbohydrates: 5-10g

Tips:

- For a more flavorful chicken, marinate it in your favorite Italian dressing for 30 minutes before grilling.
- If you don't have a grill, you can bake the skewers in the oven at 400°F for 15-20 minutes.
- To make this recipe even more filling, serve it with a side of quinoa or brown rice.
- Feel free to get creative with the ingredients! You can add other vegetables like zucchini or bell peppers, or use different types of cheese like feta or goat cheese.

Turkey and Vegetable Lettuce Wraps

COOKING TIME: 15 MINUTES | PREP TIME: 10 MINUTES | TOTAL TIME: 25 MINUTES | SERVING SIZE: 2 LETTUCE WRAPS

Ingredients:

- 4 large romaine lettuce leaves, washed and patted dry
- 4 ounces ground turkey breast
- 1/2 cup chopped red bell pepper
- 1/2 cup chopped green bell pepper
- 1/4 cup chopped onion
- 1 clove garlic, minced
- 1/4 cup low-sodium chicken broth
- 2 tablespoons soy sauce
- 1 tablespoon rice vinegar
- 1 teaspoon sesame oil
- 1/2 teaspoon sriracha (optional)
- Salt and pepper to taste

Directions:

1. In a large skillet over medium heat, cook the ground turkey until browned. Drain any excess fat.
2. Add the bell peppers, onion, and garlic to the skillet and cook until softened, about 5 minutes.
3. Stir in the chicken broth, soy sauce, rice vinegar, sesame oil, and sriracha (if using). Season with salt and pepper to taste.
4. Bring the mixture to a simmer and cook for 2-3 minutes.
5. To assemble the lettuce wraps, spoon the turkey and vegetable mixture into the romaine lettuce leaves.
6. Serve immediately.

Nutritional information (per serving): Calories: 250, Protein: 25g, Carbs: 10g, Fat: 10g

Tips:

- You can use any type of ground poultry you like, such as chicken or turkey.
- Feel free to add other vegetables to the wraps, such as carrots, mushrooms, or zucchini.
- If you don't have romaine lettuce, you can use iceberg lettuce or butter lettuce.
- For a spicier wrap, add more sriracha or red pepper flakes.
- Serve the wraps with a side of low-fat yogurt or hummus for added protein and creaminess.

Spinach and Feta Stuffed Chicken Breast

COOKING TIME: 20 MINUTES | PREP TIME: 10 MINUTES | TOTAL TIME: 30 MINUTES | SERVING SIZE: 1

Ingredients:

- 1 boneless, skinless chicken breast
- 1/2 cup chopped fresh spinach
- 1/4 cup crumbled feta cheese
- 1/4 teaspoon dried oregano
- 1/4 teaspoon garlic powder
- Salt and pepper to taste
- 1 tablespoon olive oil

Directions:

1. Preheat oven to 400°F (200°C).
2. Butterfly the chicken breast by carefully slicing it horizontally almost all the way through, leaving the hinge intact. Open the chicken breast like a book.
3. In a small bowl, combine the spinach, feta cheese, oregano, garlic powder, salt, and pepper.
4. Spread the spinach and feta mixture over the inside of the chicken breast.
5. Fold the chicken breast closed and secure the edges with toothpicks.
6. Heat the olive oil in an oven-safe skillet over medium heat. Sear the chicken breast for 2-3 minutes per side, until golden brown.
7. Transfer the skillet to the oven and bake for 15-20 minutes, or until the chicken is cooked through and the juices run clear.
8. Remove from the oven and let cool slightly before serving.

Nutritional Information (per serving): Calories: 250, Protein: 35g, Fat: 10g, Carbohydrates: 5g, Fiber: 2g

Broccoli and Cheddar Soup

COOKING TIME: 20 MINUTES | PREP TIME: 10 MINUTES | TOTAL TIME: 30 MINUTES
SERVING SIZE: 1 CUP

Ingredients:

- 1 tablespoon olive oil
- 1 onion, chopped
- 2 cloves garlic, minced
- 4 cups low-sodium chicken broth
- 2 cups broccoli florets
- 1 medium potato, peeled and diced
- 1/2 cup non-fat Greek yogurt
- 1/2 cup shredded sharp cheddar cheese
- Salt and pepper to taste

Directions:

1. Heat olive oil in a large pot over medium heat. Add onion and cook until softened, about 5 minutes.
2. Add garlic and cook for 1 minute more.
3. Add chicken broth, broccoli, and potato. Bring to a boil, then reduce heat and simmer for 15 minutes, or until vegetables are tender.
4. Using an immersion blender or blender, puree the soup until smooth.
5. Stir in Greek yogurt and cheddar cheese. Season with salt and pepper to taste.
6. Serve hot, garnished with additional cheese or a sprinkle of red pepper flakes, if desired.

Nutritional Information (per serving): Calories: 180, Protein: 15g, Fat: 8g, Carbohydrates: 15g, Fiber: 5g

Tips:

- For a lighter soup, use skim milk instead of Greek yogurt.
- You can also add other vegetables to the soup, such as carrots, celery, or zucchini.
- This soup can be frozen in individual portions for quick and easy lunches.
- To make this soup ahead of time, simply reheat it gently on the stovetop or in the microwave.

Greek Yogurt Chicken Salad

COOKING TIME: 15 MINUTES (for poaching chicken) | PREP TIME: 10 MINUTES | TOTAL TIME: 25 MINUTES | SERVING SIZE: 1 CUP

Ingredients:

- 1 boneless, skinless chicken breast (4 oz)
- 1/2 cup nonfat plain Greek yogurt
- 1/4 cup diced celery
- 1/4 cup chopped red onion
- 1/4 cup chopped apple (optional)
- 1 tablespoon fresh dill, chopped (or another herb of your choice)
- 1/2 teaspoon lemon juice
- 1/4 teaspoon Dijon mustard
- Salt and pepper to taste

Directions:

1. Poach the chicken: Fill a saucepan with water and bring to a simmer. Add the chicken breast and cook for 15 minutes, or until cooked through. Remove from the heat and let cool slightly.
2. Shred the chicken: Use two forks to shred the chicken into bite-sized pieces.
3. Combine ingredients: In a large bowl, combine the shredded chicken, Greek yogurt, celery, red onion, apple (if using), dill, lemon juice, Dijon mustard, salt, and pepper. Mix well to combine.
4. Chill and serve: Cover the bowl and refrigerate for at least 30 minutes to allow the flavors to meld. Serve on bed of lettuce, whole-wheat crackers, or as a filling for lettuce wraps.

Nutritional Information (per serving): Calories: 250, Protein: 35g, Carbs: 15g (6g fiber), fat: 5g

Tips:

- For a vegetarian option, you can replace the chicken with crumbled tofu or chickpeas.
- To add more flavor, try using other herbs like parsley, tarragon, or chives.
- You can also add additional vegetables like chopped cucumber, bell pepper, or carrots.
- If you find the salad too thick, you can add a little bit of water or chicken broth to thin it out.

Mexican Cauliflower Rice Bowl

COOKING TIME: 20 MINUTES | PREP TIME: 10 MINUTES | TOTAL TIME: 30 MINUTES | SERVING SIZE: 1 BOWL

Ingredients:

- 1 tablespoon olive oil
- 1/2 onion, diced
- 1 clove garlic, minced
- 1 cup rice cauliflower (fresh or frozen)
- 1/2 cup black beans, rinsed and drained
- 4 ounces lean ground beef, chicken, or turkey
- 1/2 teaspoon chili powder
- 1/4 teaspoon cumin
- Salt and pepper to taste
- Optional toppings: chopped cilantro, avocado slices, salsa, Greek yogurt, shredded cheese

Instructions:

1. Heat olive oil in a skillet over medium heat. Add onion and garlic, and cook until softened, about 5 minutes.

2. Add rice cauliflower and cook for another 5 minutes, stirring occasionally.

3. Stir in black beans and cook for 1 minute.

4. Add ground meat and cook until browned, breaking it up with a spoon.

5. Season with chili powder, cumin, salt, and pepper.

6. Serve the cauliflower rice mixture in a bowl and top with your desired toppings. Enjoy!

Nutritional Information (per serving): Calories: 350, Protein: 25g, Carbohydrates: 25g (8g net carbs), fat: 10g, Fiber: 8g

Tips:

- For a vegetarian option, use crumbled tofu or tempeh instead of meat.
- You can also add other vegetables to the bowl, such as corn, bell peppers, or zucchini.
- If you don't have riced cauliflower, you can grate a head of cauliflower using the pulse function of a food processor.
- Leftovers can be stored in an airtight container in the refrigerator for up to 3 days.

Lemon Garlic Shrimp Stir-Fry

COOKING TIME: 10 MINUTES | PREP TIME: 10 MINUTES | TOTAL TIME: 20 MINUTES | SERVING SIZE: 1

Ingredients:

- 4 ounces raw shrimp, peeled and deveined
- 1 tablespoon olive oil
- 1/2 cup bell peppers (any color), sliced
- 1/2 cup broccoli florets
- 1/4 cup zucchini, sliced
- 1/4 cup chicken broth
- 1 tablespoon lemon juice
- 1 clove garlic, minced
- 1/2 teaspoon dried oregano
- 1/4 teaspoon salt
- 1/4 teaspoon black pepper
- Cooked brown rice or quinoa (optional)

Directions:

1. Heat olive oil in a large skillet or wok over medium-high heat. Add shrimp and cook for 2-3 minutes per side, or until pink and cooked through. Remove from pan and set aside.
2. Add bell peppers, broccoli, and zucchini to the pan and cook for 5-7 minutes, or until tender-crisp.
3. Stir in chicken broth, lemon juice, garlic, oregano, salt, and pepper. Bring to a simmer and cook for 1 minute.
4. Return shrimp to the pan and heat through.
5. Serve over cooked brown rice or quinoa, if desired.

Nutritional Information per Serving: Calories: 300, Protein: 25g, Carbohydrates: 20g, Fat: 10g

Tips:

- You can use frozen shrimp to save time. Just thaw them in the refrigerator before cooking.
- Add other vegetables to the stir-fry, such as snap peas, carrots, or mushrooms.
- If you don't have chicken broth, you can use water or vegetable broth.
- Adjust the seasonings to your taste.

Sweet Potato and Black Bean Salad

COOKING TIME: 25 MINUTES | PREP TIME: 15 MINUTES | TOTAL TIME: 40 MINUTES | SERVING SIZE: 1

Ingredients:

- 1 medium sweet potato, peeled and cubed
- 1/2 cup black beans, rinsed and drained
- 1/4 cup red bell pepper, chopped
- 1/4 cup corn kernels (fresh or frozen)
- 1/4 cup chopped red onion
- 1/4 cup chopped cilantro
- 2 tablespoons olive oil
- 1 tablespoon lime juice
- 1/2 teaspoon chili powder
- 1/4 teaspoon cumin
- Pinch of salt and pepper

Directions:

1. Preheat oven to 400°F (200°C). Line a baking sheet with parchment paper.
2. Toss sweet potato cubes with 1 tablespoon olive oil, salt, and pepper. Spread on the prepared baking sheet and roast for 20-25 minutes, or until tender and slightly browned.
3. While the sweet potatoes roast, prepare the dressing. In a small bowl, whisk together lime juice, remaining olive oil, chili powder, cumin, salt, and pepper.
4. Once roasted, let the sweet potatoes cool slightly. In a large bowl, combine sweet potatoes, black beans, red pepper, corn, red onion, and cilantro. Pour in the dressing and toss gently to coat all ingredients.
5. Enjoy the salad immediately as is, or chill in the refrigerator for 30 minutes for deeper flavors.

Nutritional Information (Per serving): Calories: 250, Carbohydrates: 35g (net), Protein: 15g, Fat: 7g, Fiber: 8g, Iron: 4mg

Tomato Basil Mozzarella Stacks

COOKING TIME: N/A | PREP TIME: 10 MINUTES | TOTAL TIME: 10 MINUTES | SERVING SIZE: 1 STACK

Ingredients:

- 1 medium tomato, thinly sliced
- 4 Oz fresh mozzarella cheese, sliced
- 5-6 large basil leaves
- 1 tablespoon olive oil
- 1/2 teaspoon balsamic vinegar
- Pinch of salt and black pepper

Directions:

1. Assemble the stacks: Arrange 3-4 tomato slices on a plate. Top each slice with a basil leaf and a mozzarella slice. Repeat one more time, forming a stack of 3 tomato slices, 3 basil leaves, and 3 mozzarella slices.
2. Drizzle and season: Drizzle each stack with 1/2 teaspoon olive oil and 1/4 teaspoon balsamic vinegar. Season with salt and pepper to taste.
3. Serve immediately: Enjoy these stacks fresh for maximum flavor and nutritional value.

Nutritional Information per Serving: Calories: 180, Protein: 12g, Carbs: 14g (8g net carbs), fat: 8g, Fiber: 3g

Tips:

- For added variety, use different types of tomatoes, such as cherry tomatoes or heirloom varieties.
- If you're feeling fancy, drizzle the stacks with a balsamic glaze instead of balsamic vinegar.
- Add a sprinkle of fresh herbs like oregano or thyme for extra flavor.
- Serve these stacks alongside a side salad with a light vinaigrette dressing for a complete and balanced meal.

Mushroom and Spinach Stuffed Bell Peppers

COOKING TIME: 25 MINUTES | PREP TIME: 15 MINUTES | TOTAL TIME: 40 MINUTES | SERVING SIZE: 2

Ingredients:

- 2 bell peppers (any color)
- 1 tablespoon olive oil
- 1/2 onion, diced
- 2 cloves garlic, minced
- 8 ounces mushrooms, sliced
- 5 ounces fresh spinach, chopped (or 10 ounces frozen, thawed)
- 1/2 teaspoon dried oregano
- 1/4 teaspoon salt
- 1/4 teaspoon black pepper
- 1/4 cup low-fat ricotta cheese
- 1/4 cup shredded low-fat mozzarella cheese
- Fresh parsley, chopped (optional)

Instructions:

1. Preheat oven to 375°F (190°C).
2. Halve the bell peppers, removing the seeds and membranes. Place them in a baking dish, cut-side up.
3. Heat olive oil in a skillet over medium heat. Add onion and cook until softened, about 5 minutes.
4. Add garlic and mushrooms, cook until browned, about 5 minutes more.
5. Stir in spinach, oregano, salt, and pepper. Cook until spinach is wilted, about 2 minutes.
6. Divide the mushroom mixture evenly between the bell pepper halves.
7. Top with ricotta cheese and sprinkle with mozzarella cheese.
8. Bake for 25 minutes, or until the peppers are tender and the cheese is melted.
9. Garnish with fresh parsley, if desired.

Nutritional Information (per serving): Calories: 200, Protein: 15g, Carbohydrates: 15g, Fiber: 5g, Fat: 5g

Turkey and Cranberry Lettuce Wraps

COOKING TIME: 5 MINUTES (IF USING LEFTOVER TURKEY OR CHICKEN) | PREP TIME: 10 MINUTES | TOTAL TIME: 15 MINUTES | SERVING SIZE: 2 WRAPS

Ingredients:

- 4 large romaine lettuce leaves, washed and patted dry
- 4 Oz cooked and shredded turkey or chicken breast (grilled, roasted, or poached)
- 2 tbsp. cranberry sauce (low-sugar preferred)
- 1/4 cup crumbled feta cheese
- 1/4 cup chopped walnuts
- Salt and pepper to taste

Optional Garnishes:

- Sliced avocado
- Chopped fresh herbs (cilantro, parsley, chives)
- Dijon mustard
- Greek yogurt

Directions:

1. Assemble the wraps: Place a romaine lettuce leaf on a plate. Spread 1 tbsp. of cranberry sauce onto the leaf.
2. Add the protein: Top with 2 Oz of cooked and shredded turkey or chicken.
3. Layer the toppings: Sprinkle with feta cheese, walnuts, salt, and pepper to taste.
4. Wrap it up: Fold the sides of the lettuce leaf over the filling and roll up tightly
5. Repeat: Assemble the remaining wraps and enjoy!

Nutritional Information (per wrap): Calories: 250, Protein: 30g, Carbohydrates: 5g, Fat: 10g

Asian-Inspired Chicken and Vegetable Skewers

COOKING TIME: 10-12 MINUTES| PREP TIME: 15 MINUTES | TOTAL TIME: 25-27 MINUTES | SERVING SIZE: 2 SKEWERS (1 SERVING)

Ingredients:

- 4 Oz boneless, skinless chicken breast, cubed
- 1/2 cup bell pepper (any color), chopped
- 1/2 cup zucchini, chopped
- 1/4 cup red onion, chopped
- 1/4 cup low-sodium soy sauce
- 1 tbsp. rice vinegar
- 1 tbsp. sriracha (adjust for spice preference)
- 1 tsp. grated ginger
- 1/2 tsp. sesame oil
- 1/4 tsp. garlic powder
- 1/4 tsp. black pepper
- Wooden skewers (soaked for at least 30 minutes to prevent burning)

Directions:

1. Combine marinade: In a bowl, whisk together soy sauce, rice vinegar, sriracha, ginger, sesame oil, garlic powder, and black pepper.
2. Marinate chicken: Add the chicken cubes to the marinade and toss to coat. Cover and refrigerate for at least 15 minutes, or up to 2 hours for deeper flavor.
3. Prepare vegetables: While the chicken marinates, chop the bell pepper, zucchini, and red onion.
4. Assemble skewers: Thread the chicken and vegetables onto skewers, alternating between protein and veggies for even cooking.
5. Cook: Preheat your grill or grill pan to medium-high heat. Grill the skewers for 10-12 minutes per side, or until the chicken is cooked through and the vegetables are tender-crisp.
6. Serve: Enjoy your skewers warm with a side of brown rice or a mixed green salad.

Nutritional Information (per serving): Calories: 250-300, Protein: 30-35g, Fat: 5-7g, Carbohydrates: 15-20g, Fiber: 3-5g

DINNER RECIPES

Baked Lemon Herb Chicken

COOKING TIME: 20-25 MINUTES | PREP TIME: 10 MINUTES | TOTAL TIME: 30-35 MINUTES | SERVING SIZE: 1 CHICKEN BREAST

Ingredients:

- 1 boneless, skinless chicken breast (4-5 Oz)
- 1/4 cup lemon juice (freshly squeezed is best)
- 1 tablespoon olive oil
- 1/2 teaspoon dried oregano
- 1/2 teaspoon dried thyme
- 1/4 teaspoon salt
- 1/4 teaspoon black pepper
- 1/4 cup chopped fresh parsley (optional)

Directions:

1. Preheat oven to 400°F (200°C).
2. In a small bowl, whisk together lemon juice, olive oil, oregano, thyme, salt, and pepper.
3. Place the chicken breast in a shallow baking dish. Pour the marinade over the chicken, ensuring it is coated evenly.
4. Bake for 20-25 minutes, or until the chicken is cooked through and juices run clear. An internal temperature of 165°F (74°C) is recommended.
5. Garnish with fresh parsley (optional) and serve immediately.

Nutritional Information (per serving): Calories: 250, Protein: 35g, Fat: 5g, Carbohydrates: 5g, Fiber: 1g

Cauliflower Crust Pizza

COOKING TIME: 25 MINUTES | PREP TIME: 15 MINUTES |TOTAL TIME: 40 MINUTES | SERVING SIZE: 1 SMALL PIZZA (1/2 recipe)

Ingredients:

- 1 head cauliflower, chopped
- 1 egg
- 1/2 cup shredded mozzarella cheese
- 1/4 cup grated Parmesan cheese
- 1/2 teaspoon Italian seasoning
- 1/4 teaspoon garlic powder
- 1/4 teaspoon onion powder
- Salt and pepper to taste
- 1/4 cup low-sugar marinara sauce
- 1/4 cup chopped vegetables (bell peppers, mushrooms, onions)
- 1 ounce lean protein (cooked chicken, turkey, ground beef) (optional)

Directions:

1. Preheat oven to 400°F (200°C). Line a baking sheet with parchment paper.
2. Pulse cauliflower in a food processor until finely grated. Alternatively, use a box grater.
3. Place the cauliflower in a microwave-safe bowl and microwave for 5-7 minutes. Drain any excess moisture with a clean kitchen towel.
4. Transfer the cauliflower to a mixing bowl and add the egg, mozzarella cheese, Parmesan cheese, Italian seasoning, garlic powder, onion powder, salt, and pepper. Mix well until well combined.
5. Spread the cauliflower mixture into a 10-inch circle on the prepared baking sheet. Press down firmly to form a compact crust.
6. Bake for 20-25 minutes, or until golden brown and crispy.
7. Spread the marinara sauce evenly over the crust. Top with your favorite vegetables and optional protein.
8. Return the pizza to the oven and broil for 2-3 minutes, or until the cheese is melted and bubbly.
9. Let cool slightly before slicing and serving.

Nutritional Information per Serving: Calories: 250, Carbohydrates: 15g (net), Protein: 20g, Fat: 10g

Shrimp and Veggie Stir-Fry

COOKING TIME: 10-12 MINUTES | PREP TIME: 5 MINUTES | TOTAL TIME: 15-17 MINUTES | SERVING SIZE: 1 CUP

Ingredients:

- 4 ounces raw shrimp, peeled and deveined (frozen, thawed shrimp works great)
- 1 cup broccoli florets
- 1 cup bell pepper strips (red, yellow, or orange)
- 1/2 cup snow peas
- 1/4 cup sliced onion
- 1 clove garlic, minced
- 1 tablespoon low-sodium soy sauce
- 1 tablespoon rice vinegar
- 1 teaspoon cornstarch
- 1/2 teaspoon sesame oil
- 1/4 teaspoon ground ginger
- Pinch of black pepper
- Freshly chopped scallions, for garnish (optional)

Directions:

1. Prep the Vegetables: Wash and chop all the vegetables to desired sizes.
2. Marinate the Shrimp: In a bowl, combine the shrimp with cornstarch, sesame oil, ginger, and black pepper. Mix well and set aside for 5 minutes.
3. Cook the Shrimp: Heat a large wok or skillet over medium-high heat. Add 1 teaspoon of oil and swirl to coat the bottom. Add the marinated shrimp and cook for 2-3 minutes per side, or until pink and cooked through. Remove from the pan and set aside.
4. Stir-Fry the Vegetables: Add the remaining oil to the wok or skillet. Add the onion and cook for 1 minute, until softened. Then, add the bell peppers and broccoli, and stir-fry for 3-4 minutes, or until slightly tender-crisp.
5. Make the Sauce: In a small bowl, whisk together the soy sauce, rice vinegar, cornstarch, and a pinch of black pepper.
6. Finish the Stir-Fry: Pour the sauce into the wok with the vegetables and let it simmer for 1 minute, until slightly thickened. Add the cooked shrimp back to the pan and stir to combine.
7. Serve and Garnish: Immediately transfer the stir-fry to a plate and serve hot. Garnish with chopped scallions, if desired.

Nutritional Information (per Serving): Calories: 250-270, Protein: 20-25 grams, Carbohydrates: 15-20 grams (mostly from vegetables), fat: 5-7 grams, Fiber: 2-3 grams

Turkey and Vegetable Meatballs

COOKING TIME: 20-25 MINUTES| PREP TIME: 10 MINUTES | TOTAL TIME: 30 MINUTES | SERVING SIZE: 6 MEATBALLS (1 SERVING)

Ingredients:

- 1 pound ground turkey (90% lean or higher)
- 1/2 cup finely chopped mixed vegetables (carrots, zucchini, onion, celery)
- 1/2 cup panko breadcrumbs
- 1/4 cup chopped fresh parsley
- 1 egg, beaten
- 1 tablespoon Dijon mustard
- 1 teaspoon dried oregano
- 1/2 teaspoon garlic powder
- 1/4 teaspoon salt
- 1/4 teaspoon black pepper

Directions:

1. Preheat oven to 400°F (200°C). Line a baking sheet with parchment paper.

2. In a large bowl, combine ground turkey, chopped vegetables, breadcrumbs, parsley, egg, Dijon mustard, oregano, garlic powder, salt, and pepper. Mix well until evenly combined.

3. Roll the mixture into 12 equal-sized meatballs.

4. Place the meatballs on the prepared baking sheet.

5. Bake for 20-25 minutes, or until the meatballs are cooked through and golden brown.

6. Serve immediately with your favorite marinara sauce, roasted vegetables, or a side salad.

Nutritional Information (per Serving): Calories: 180, Protein: 25g, Fat: 5g, Carbohydrates: 10g, Fiber: 2g

Salmon and Asparagus Foil Packets

COOKING TIME: 15-20 MINUTES | PREP TIME: 10 MINUTES | TOTAL TIME: 25-30 MINUTES | SERVING SIZE: 1 PACKET

Ingredients:

- 4 (4-ounce) salmon fillets
- 1 pound asparagus, trimmed
- 1 tablespoon olive oil
- 1/2 lemon, sliced
- 1/4 teaspoon dried thyme
- Salt and pepper to taste

- **Optional additions:**
- 1 clove garlic, minced
- 1 tablespoon chopped fresh parsley
- 1 teaspoon Dijon mustard
- 1/4 teaspoon red pepper flakes

Directions:

1. Preheat oven to 400°F (200°C).
2. Lay out four squares of aluminum foil large enough to enclose the salmon and asparagus.
3. Brush each foil square with olive oil.
4. Place a salmon fillet in the center of each foil square.
5. Top each salmon fillet with asparagus spears, lemon slices, and thyme.
6. Season with salt and pepper to taste.
7. If using, add garlic, parsley, Dijon mustard, and red pepper flakes (optional).
8. Fold the foil edges up and over the salmon and asparagus, crimping the edges to seal the packets.
9. Place the packets on a baking sheet.
10. Bake for 15-20 minutes, or until the salmon is cooked through and the asparagus is tender-crisp.
11. Carefully open the packets and serve immediately.

Nutritional Information (per serving): Calories: 250-300, Protein: 30-35g, Fat: 10-15g, Carbohydrates: 5-10g

Baked Zucchini Boats

COOKING TIME: 15-20 MINUTES | PREP TIME: 10 MINUTES | TOTAL TIME: 25-30 MINUTES | SERVING SIZE: 1

Ingredients:

- 2 medium zucchini
- 1/2 pound lean ground turkey or chicken breast
- 1/2 cup diced onion
- 1/2 cup chopped mushrooms
- 1/4 cup low-sugar marinara sauce
- 1/4 cup shredded low-fat mozzarella cheese
- 1/4 teaspoon Italian seasoning
- Salt and pepper to taste

Directions:

1. Preheat oven to 400°F (200°C).
2. Cut the zucchini in half lengthwise and scoop out the flesh, leaving a 1/2-inch border. Set the flesh aside.
3. Place the zucchini halves in a baking dish, cut side up.
4. In a medium skillet, cook the ground turkey or chicken over medium heat until browned. Drain any excess fat.
5. Add the onion and mushrooms to the skillet and cook until softened, about 5 minutes.
6. Stir in the marinara sauce, Italian seasoning, salt, and pepper.
7. Spoon the turkey mixture into the zucchini boats.
8. Top with shredded cheese.
9. Bake for 15-20 minutes, or until the zucchini is tender and the cheese is melted and bubbly.

Nutritional Information (per serving): Calories: 150-200, Protein: 15-20g, Carbohydrates: 10-15g, Fat: 5-10g, Fiber: 3-5g

Chicken and Broccoli Casserole

PREPARATION TIME: 15 MINUTES | COOKING TIME: 30 MINUTES | TOTAL TIME: 45 MINUTES | SERVING SIZE: 1 SERVING

Ingredients:

- 4 Oz boneless, skinless chicken breast, diced
- 1 cup frozen broccoli florets, thawed
- 1/2 cup fat-free chicken broth
- 1/4 cup nonfat Greek yogurt
- 1/4 cup shredded low-fat mozzarella cheese
- 1/4 teaspoon dried thyme
- 1/4 teaspoon garlic powder
- Salt and pepper to taste

Directions:

1. Preheat oven to 375°F (190°C). Spray a small baking dish with nonstick cooking spray.
2. In a bowl, combine the chicken, broccoli, chicken broth, Greek yogurt, mozzarella cheese, thyme, garlic powder, salt, and pepper. Mix well to coat the chicken and broccoli evenly.
3. Transfer the mixture to the prepared baking dish. Spread it out evenly in a single layer.
4. Bake for 30 minutes, or until the chicken is cooked through and the sauce is bubbly.
5. Let cool slightly before serving.

Nutritional Information (per serving): Calories: 250, Protein: 35g, Fat: 5g, Carbohydrates: 15g

Tips:

- You can use other vegetables in place of broccoli, such as cauliflower, zucchini, or bell peppers.
- For a richer flavor, add a tablespoon of grated Parmesan cheese before baking.
- If you prefer a thicker sauce, mix 1 tablespoon of cornstarch with 2 tablespoons of cold water and stir into the chicken mixture before baking.
- Serve this casserole with a side of brown rice or quinoa for a complete meal.

Eggplant Lasagna

COOKING TIME: 45 MINUTES | PREP TIME: 20 MINUTES | TOTAL TIME: 65 MINUTES | SERVING SIZE: 1

Ingredients:

- 1 medium eggplant, thinly sliced
- 1 tablespoon olive oil
- 1/2 teaspoon dried oregano
- 1/4 teaspoon salt
- 1/4 teaspoon black pepper
- 1 (15-ounce) can diced tomatoes, undrained
- 1/2 cup low-fat ricotta cheese
- 1/4 cup grated Parmesan cheese
- 1/4 cup chopped fresh basil

Directions:

1. Preheat oven to 400°F (200°C).
2. Prep the eggplant: Brush both sides of each eggplant slice with olive oil, sprinkle with oregano, salt, and pepper. Lay slices on a baking sheet in a single layer and bake for 15 minutes, flipping halfway through, until tender and lightly browned.
3. Assemble the lasagna: In a small bowl, mix diced tomatoes with a pinch of salt and pepper. Spread a thin layer of tomato sauce in the bottom of a small baking dish (approximately 6x8 inches). Top with 1/3 of the baked eggplant slices, then 1/3 of the ricotta cheese, and sprinkle with 1/2 tablespoon of Parmesan cheese. Repeat with another layer of tomato sauce, eggplant, ricotta, and Parmesan. Finish with the remaining tomato sauce and Parmesan cheese.
4. Bake: Cover the dish with foil and bake for 30 minutes. Uncover and bake for an additional 10 minutes, or until bubbly and golden brown.
5. Serve: Let the lasagna cool slightly before slicing and serving. Garnish with chopped fresh basil for an extra flavor boost.

Nutritional Information (per serving): Calories: 350, Carbohydrates: 25g (10g net carbs), Protein: 30g, Fat: 15g

Quinoa-Stuffed Peppers

COOKING TIME: 35 MINUTES | PREP TIME: 15 MINUTES | TOTAL TIME: 50 MINUTES | SERVING SIZE: 2

Ingredients:

- 2 bell peppers (any color)
- 1/2 cup uncooked quinoa, rinsed
- 1 cup vegetable broth
- 1/2 pound lean ground turkey
- 1/2 onion, diced
- 1 clove garlic, minced
- 1/2 cup chopped mushrooms
- 1/2 cup chopped zucchini
- 1/4 cup chopped sun-dried tomatoes
- 1/4 cup chopped fresh parsley
- 1/2 teaspoon dried oregano
- 1/4 teaspoon smoked paprika
- Salt and pepper to tast

Instructions:

1. Preheat oven to 375°F (190°C).

2. Cut the bell peppers in half lengthwise and remove the seeds and membranes. Place the peppers cut-side up in a baking dish.

3. In a saucepan, combine the quinoa and vegetable broth. Bring to a boil, then reduce heat, cover, and simmer for 15 minutes or until the quinoa is cooked and fluffy.

4. While the quinoa is cooking, heat olive oil in a skillet over medium heat. Add the ground turkey and cook until browned, breaking it up with a spoon.

5. Add the onion, garlic, mushrooms, and zucchini to the pan and cook until softened, about 5 minutes.

6. Stir in the cooked quinoa, sun-dried tomatoes, parsley, oregano, paprika, salt, and pepper. Mix well to combine.

7. Spoon the quinoa mixture into the bell pepper halves.

8. Bake for 35 minutes, or until the peppers are tender and the filling is heated through.

9. Serve immediately and enjoy!

Nutritional information (per serving): Calories: 300, Protein: 25g, Carbohydrates: 25g (net carbs), fat: 10g

Ach Stuffed Mushrooms

PREP TIME: 15 MINUTES | COOKING TIME: 15-20 MINUTES | TOTAL TIME: 30-35 MINUTES | SERVING SIZE: This recipe makes 6 servings, with each serving being 1 large Portobello mushroom cap.

Ingredients:

- 6 large Portobello mushroom caps
- 1 (14 Oz) can artichoke hearts, drained and chopped
- ½ cup chopped spinach
- ¼ cup ricotta cheese
- 2 cloves garlic, minced
- ½ cup shredded Parmesan cheese
- ¼ cup chopped fresh parsley
- Salt and pepper to taste

Directions:

1. Preheat oven to 375°F (190°C).
2. Gently remove the stems from the Portobello mushrooms and clean the caps with a damp paper towel.
3. In a medium bowl, combine chopped artichoke hearts, spinach, ricotta cheese, garlic, Parmesan cheese, and parsley. Season with salt and pepper to taste.
4. Spoon the artichoke mixture evenly into the portobello mushroom caps.
5. Place the stuffed mushrooms on a baking sheet lined with parchment paper.
6. Bake for 15-20 minutes, or until the mushrooms are tender and the filling is bubbly.
7. Serve immediately.

Nutritional Information (per serving): Calories: 150, Protein: 12g, Carbs: 5g, Fat: 8g, Fiber: 3g

Vegetable and Chicken Skewers

COOKING TIME: 15-20 MINUTES | PREP TIME: 10 MINUTES | TOTAL TIME: 25-30 MINUTES | SERVING SIZE: 2 SKEWERS (1 SERVING)

Ingredients:

- 4 Oz boneless, skinless chicken breast, cut into cubes
- 1/2 bell pepper, cut into chunks
- 1/2 zucchini, cut into chunks
- 1/4 red onion, cut into wedges
- 1 tablespoon olive oil
- 1/2 teaspoon dried oregano
- 1/4 teaspoon garlic powder
- 1/4 teaspoon salt
- 1/4 teaspoon black pepper
- 8 bamboo skewers

Directions:

1. Preheat oven to 400°F (200°C).
2. In a large bowl, combine chicken, bell pepper, zucchini, and red onion.
3. In a small bowl, whisk together olive oil, oregano, garlic powder, salt, and pepper. Pour over the chicken and vegetables and toss to coat.
4. Thread the chicken and vegetables onto skewers.
5. Arrange the skewers on a baking sheet lined with parchment paper.
6. Bake for 15-20 minutes, or until the chicken is cooked through and the vegetables are tender.
7. Serve immediately.

Nutritional information (per serving): Calories: 250, Protein: 30g, Fat: 5g, Carbohydrates: 15g, Fiber: 2g

Zoodle (Zucchini Noodle) Stir-Fry

COOKING TIME: 15 MINUTES | PREP TIME: 10 MINUTES | TOTAL TIME: 25 MINUTES | SERVING SIZE: 1

Ingredients:

- 2 tablespoons olive oil
- 1 red bell pepper, thinly sliced
- 1 onion, thinly sliced
- 2 cloves garlic, minced
- 1 pound zucchini, spiralized
- 1 cup shredded lean chicken breast or tofu
- 1/2 cup low-sodium chicken broth
- 2 tablespoons low-sodium soy sauce
- 1 tablespoon rice vinegar
- 1 teaspoon sesame oil
- 1/2 teaspoon crushed red pepper flakes (optional)
- Freshly ground black pepper, to taste
- Sesame seeds and chopped green onions, for garnish (optional)

Directions:

1. Heat olive oil in a large wok or skillet over medium heat. Add bell pepper and onion, and cook for 5 minutes, or until softened.
2. Stir in garlic and cook for 30 seconds until fragrant.
3. Add spiralized zucchini and cook for 3-5 minutes, stirring occasionally, until tender-crisp.
4. Add chicken or tofu and cook for 1-2 minutes, until warmed through.
5. In a small bowl, whisk together chicken broth, soy sauce, rice vinegar, sesame oil, and red pepper flakes (if using). Pour the sauce into the pan and stir to combine.
6. Cook for 1 minute, then season with black pepper to taste.
7. Serve immediately, garnished with sesame seeds and chopped green onions (optional).

Nutritional Information (per serving): Calories: 250, Carbohydrates: 15g (net), Protein: 20g, Fat: 10g, Fiber: 5g

Lemon Garlic Grilled Chicken Thighs

COOKING TIME: 15-20 MINUTES | PREP TIME: 10 MINUTES | TOTAL TIME: 25-30 MINUTES | SERVING SIZE: 1 CHICKEN THIGH (4 OZ)

Ingredients:

- 2 boneless, skinless chicken thighs (about 4 Oz each)
- 1 tablespoon olive oil
- 1 tablespoon lemon juice
- 1 clove garlic, minced
- 1/2 teaspoon dried oregano
- 1/4 teaspoon dried thyme
- Salt and pepper to taste

Directions:

1. Preheat your grill to medium heat.
2. In a small bowl, whisk together olive oil, lemon juice, garlic, oregano, thyme, salt, and pepper.
3. Place the chicken thighs in a shallow dish and pour the marinade over them. Toss to coat evenly.
4. Marinate for at least 10 minutes, or up to 30 minutes for deeper flavor.
5. Place the chicken thighs on the preheated grill and cook for 7-8 minutes per side, or until cooked through and an internal temperature of 165°F is reached.
6. Serve immediately with your favorite bariatric-friendly sides, such as roasted vegetables, quinoa, or brown rice.

Nutritional Information (per serving): Calories: 220, Protein: 35g, Fat: 8g, Carbohydrates: 1g

Tips:

- For added smoky flavor, soak some wood chips in water for 30 minutes before grilling and toss them on the coals just before placing the chicken on the grill.
- If you don't have a grill, you can cook the chicken in a grill pan over medium heat.
- Leftover chicken can be stored in an airtight container in the refrigerator for up to 3 days.

Mushroom and Spinach Cauliflower Rice Risotto

PREP TIME: 10 MINUTES | COOK TIME: 25 MINUTES | TOTAL TIME: 35 MINUTES | SERVING SIZE: 1 CUP

Ingredients:

- 1 head cauliflower, cut into florets
- 1 tablespoon olive oil
- 1/2 onion, chopped
- 2 cloves garlic, minced
- 8 ounces mushrooms, sliced
- 1/2 cup vegetable broth
- 1/4 cup dry white wine (optional)
- 1/2 cup chopped spinach
- 1/4 cup grated Parmesan cheese
- Salt and pepper to taste

Instructions:

1. Prep the cauliflower: Pulse the cauliflower florets in a food processor until they resemble rice grains. You can also use pre-riced cauliflower to save time. [Image of Cauliflower florets pulsed in a food processor]
2. Sauté the aromatics: Heat the olive oil in a large skillet over medium heat. Add the onion and cook until softened, about 5 minutes. Add the garlic and cook for another minute, until fragrant.
3. Cook the mushrooms: Add the sliced mushrooms to the skillet and cook until browned and tender, about 5-7 minutes.
4. Add the cauliflower rice: Stir in the riced cauliflower and cook for 2-3 minutes, until slightly softened.
5. Deglaze with broth and wine (optional): Pour in the vegetable broth and white wine (if using) and scrape up any browned bits from the bottom of the pan. Let the liquid simmer until almost completely absorbed, about 5 minutes.
6. Stir in spinach and cheese: Add the chopped spinach and cook until wilted. Stir in the Parmesan cheese and season with salt and pepper to taste.
7. Serve immediately: Enjoy your warm and flavorful Mushroom and Spinach Cauliflower Rice Risotto!

Nutritional Information (per Serving): Calories: 250, Carbohydrates: 15g (net), Protein: 18g, Fat: 12g, Fiber: 4g

Caprese Stuffed Chicken Breast

COOKING TIME: 20-25 MINUTES | PREP TIME: 10 MINUTES | TOTAL TIME: 30-35 MINUTES | SERVING SIZE: 1 CHICKEN BREAST

Ingredients:

- 4 boneless, skinless chicken breasts (thinly pounded)
- 2 large vine-ripened tomatoes, thinly sliced
- 4 Oz fresh mozzarella cheese, thinly sliced
- 1/4 cup fresh basil leaves, torn
- 1/4 teaspoon dried oregano
- 1/4 teaspoon garlic powder
- Salt and pepper to taste
- 1 tablespoon olive oil

Directions:

1. Preheat oven to 400°F (200°C).
2. Place each chicken breast on a cutting board and gently butterfly it by making a horizontal cut 3/4 of the way through, without cutting all the way through. Open the chicken like a book.
3. Season both sides of the chicken with oregano, garlic powder, salt, and pepper.
4. Layer tomato slices, mozzarella slices, and basil leaves inside each chicken pocket. Fold the chicken closed and secure with 2-3 toothpicks.
5. Heat olive oil in a large oven-proof skillet over medium heat. Sear the chicken on each side for 2-3 minutes until golden brown.
6. Transfer the skillet to the preheated oven and bake for 20-25 minutes, or until the chicken is cooked through and no longer pink in the center.
7. Remove from the oven and let cool slightly before serving. Discard toothpicks.

Nutritional Information (per serving): Calories: 250, Carbohydrates: 5g, Fat: 5g, Protein: 35g

Blackened Tilapia Tacos

COOKING TIME: 5 MINUTES | PREP TIME: 10 MINUTES | TOTAL TIME: 15 MINUTES | SERVING SIZE: 2 TACOS

Ingredients:

- 2 tilapia fillets
- 1 tablespoon olive oil
- 1/2 teaspoon smoked paprika
- 1/2 teaspoon chili powder
- 1/4 teaspoon garlic powder
- 1/4 teaspoon onion powder
- 1/4 teaspoon black pepper
- 1/4 teaspoon cayenne pepper (optional)
- 2 small corn tortillas
- 1/2 cup chopped cabbage
- 1/4 cup diced avocado
- 1/4 cup salsa
- Cilantro, for garnish (optional)

Directions:

1. Preheat a grill pan or skillet over medium-high heat.
2. In a small bowl, whisk together the olive oil, paprika, chili powder, garlic powder, onion powder, black pepper, and cayenne pepper (if using).
3. Brush the tilapia fillets with the spice mixture.
4. Place the tilapia fillets in the preheated pan and cook for 3-4 minutes per side, or until cooked through.
5. While the tilapia is cooking, warm the tortillas in a dry pan or microwave for a few seconds.
6. To assemble the tacos, top each tortilla with a tilapia fillet, cabbage, avocado, and salsa. Garnish with cilantro, if desired.

Nutritional Information (per serving): Calories: 250, Fat: 5g, Carbohydrates: 15g, Protein: 30g, Fiber: 2g

Mediterranean Turkey Burgers

PREP TIME: 15 MINUTES | COOKING TIME: 10 MINUTES | TOTAL TIME: 25 MINUTES | SERVING SIZE: 1

Ingredients:

- 1 pound ground turkey (90% lean or higher)
- 1/4 cup finely chopped red onion
- 2 cloves garlic, minced
- 1/4 cup chopped sun-dried tomatoes (not oil-packed)
- 1/4 cup chopped fresh parsley
- 1 tablespoon olive oil
- 1 teaspoon dried oregano
- 1/2 teaspoon dried thyme
- 1/4 teaspoon salt
- 1/4 teaspoon black pepper
- 4 hamburger buns (whole-wheat or multigrain recommended)
- 1/2 cup sliced cucumber
- 1/4 cup crumbled feta cheese (optional)
- 1/4 cup hummus (optional)

Directions:

1. In a large bowl, combine ground turkey, red onion, garlic, sun-dried tomatoes, parsley, olive oil, oregano, thyme, salt, and pepper. Mix gently until just combined. Avoid over mixing.
2. Divide the mixture into 4 equal portions and form into patties.
3. Heat a grill pan or skillet over medium heat. Lightly coat the pan with cooking spray (optional).
4. Cook the patties for 5-7 minutes per side, or until cooked through. An internal temperature of 165°F is safe for consumption.
5. Toast the hamburger buns, if desired.
6. To assemble the burgers, place a patty on each bun bottom. Top with cucumber, feta cheese (optional), and hummus (optional). Enjoy!

Nutritional information (per serving): Calories: 250, Protein: 25g, Fat: 10g, Carbohydrates: 15g, Fiber: 2g

Cabbage and Turkey Sauté

PREP TIME: 10 MINUTES | COOK TIME: 20 MINUTES | TOTAL TIME: 30 MINUTES | SERVING SIZE: 1

Ingredients:

- 1 tablespoon olive oil
- 1/2 pound ground turkey (90% lean or higher)
- 1 small onion, diced
- 2 cloves garlic, minced
- 1/2 head green cabbage, thinly sliced
- 1/2 cup chicken broth (unsalted)
- 1/4 teaspoon dried thyme
- Salt and pepper to taste

Optional toppings:

- Chopped fresh parsley
- Sliced scallions
- Nonfat Greek yogurt
- Hot sauce

Instructions:

1. Heat olive oil in a large skillet over medium heat. Add the ground turkey and cook until browned, breaking it up with a spoon. Drain any excess fat.
2. Add the onion and garlic to the skillet and cook until softened, about 5 minutes.
3. Stir in the cabbage and chicken broth. Bring to a simmer and cook for 10-15 minutes, or until the cabbage is tender.
4. Stir in the thyme, salt, and pepper to taste.
5. Serve immediately, topped with your desired toppings.

Nutritional Information (per serving): Calories: 250, Protein: 30g, Carbs: 15g, Fat: 5gm, Fiber: 5g

Greek Yogurt with Berries

COOKING TIME: 0 MINUTES | PREP TIME: 5 MINUTES | TOTAL TIME: 5 MINUTES | SERVING SIZE: 1 CUP

Ingredients:

- 1 cup plain Greek yogurt (2% fat or non-fat)
- 1/2 cup fresh or frozen berries (blueberries, raspberries, strawberries, etc.)
- 1/4 teaspoon vanilla extract (optional)
- 1/4 cup chopped nuts or seeds (optional)

Directions:

1. In a bowl, layer half of the Greek yogurt.
2. Top with half of the berries.
3. Drizzle with a little vanilla extract, if desired.
4. Repeat with the remaining yogurt and berries.
5. Sprinkle with chopped nuts or seeds, if desired.
6. Enjoy immediately!

Nutritional information (per serving): Calories: 200, Fat: 5 grams, Carbohydrates: 15 grams, Fiber: 3 grams, Protein: 20 grams

Tips:

- For a sweeter parfait, use sweetened Greek yogurt or add a drizzle of honey or maple syrup.
- If using frozen berries, thaw them slightly before adding them to the parfait.
- Get creative with your toppings! You can also add other fruits, granola, or shredded coconut.
- Make a larger batch of the parfait and store it in the refrigerator for grab-and-go snacks throughout the week.

String Cheese and Grape Tomatoes

PREP TIME: 5 MINUTES | COOKING TIME: 0 MINUTES | TOTAL TIME: 5 MINUTES | SERVING SIZE: 1

Ingredients:

- 2 string cheese sticks
- 1/2 cup grape tomatoes

Directions:

1. Wash the grape tomatoes.
2. Cut the string cheese sticks in half (optional).
3. Place the string cheese sticks and grape tomatoes on a plate.
4. Enjoy!

Nutritional Information: Calories: 150, Protein: 12 grams, Fat: 8 grams, Carbohydrates: 8 grams, Fiber: 2 grams

Tips:

- You can use any type of cheese that you like.
- If you don't like grape tomatoes, you can use any other type of tomato or another fruit.
- You can add a sprinkle of nuts or seeds for extra protein and crunch.
- This snack is also a great option for kids.

Protein Smoothie

PREP TIME: 5 MINUTES | COOKING TIME: 0 MINUTES | TOTAL TIME: 5 MINUTES | SERVING SIZE: 1 SMOOTHIE

Ingredients:

- 1 scoop of protein powder
- 1 cup unsweetened almond milk
- 1/2 cup frozen berries
- 1/4 cup spinach
- 1/4 cup ice

Dircctions:

1. Place all ingredients in a blender and blend until smooth.
2. Pour into a glass and enjoy!

Nutritional information: Calories: 200, Protein: 25 grams, Carbohydrates: 15 grams, Fat: 5 grams, Fiber: 4 grams

Tips:

- You can use any type of protein powder that you like.
- If you don't have almond milk, you can use another type of unsweetened milk.
- You can add other fruits or vegetables to the smoothie, such as banana, mango, or kale.
- If you want to make the smoothie thicker, add more ice.
- If you want to make the smoothie thinner, add more liquid.

Cottage Cheese with Pineapple

COOKING TIME: N/A | PREP TIME: 5 MINUTES | TOTAL TIME: 5 MINUTES | SERVING SIZE: 1/2 CUP

Ingredients:

- 1/2 cup low-fat cottage cheese
- 1/4 cup chopped fresh pineapple
- 1/4 teaspoon ground cinnamon
- 1/4 teaspoon chopped fresh mint (optional)

Directions:

1. In a small bowl, combine cottage cheese and pineapple.
2. Sprinkle with cinnamon and mint (if using).
3. Stir gently to combine.
4. Serve immediately.

Nutritional Information (per serving): Calories: 150, Carbohydrates: 10g (5g from pineapple, 5g from lactose), Fiber: 2g, Protein: 15g, Fat: 2g

Tips:

- You can use canned pineapple in its own juice, but be sure to drain and rinse it well before adding it to the cottage cheese.
- For a sweeter snack, add a few drops of stevia or a drizzle of honey.
- If you don't have fresh mint, you can use a pinch of dried mint instead.
- This snack can be stored in an airtight container in the refrigerator for up to 2 days.

Almond Butter and Apple Slices

PREP TIME: 5 MINUTES | COOKING TIME: 0 MINUTES |TOTAL TIME: 5 MINUTES | SERVING SIZE: 1

Ingredients:

- 1/4 cup almond butter
- 1 apple, sliced

Directions:

1. Spread the almond butter on apple slices.
2. Enjoy!

Nutritional information: Calories: 190, Protein: 6 grams, Fiber: 4 grams, Sugar: 9 gram, Fat: 8 grams

Tips:

- You can use any type of nut butter you like, such as peanut butter or cashew butter.
- If you are not a fan of almond butter, you can try using cream cheese or hummus instead.
- For a sweeter snack, you can drizzle the apple slices with honey or maple syrup.
- You can also add other toppings to your apple slices, such as chopped nuts, seeds, or dried fruit.

Hard-Boiled Eggs

COOKING TIME: 10-12 MINUTES | PREP TIME: 5 MINUTES | TOTAL TIME: 15 MINUTES | SERVING SIZE: 1 EGG

Ingredients:

- 1 egg
- Cold water

Instructions:

1. Place the egg in a saucepan and cover it with cold water.
2. Bring the water to a boil, then reduce the heat to low and simmer for 10-12 minutes.
3. Remove the pan from the heat and let the eggs sit in the hot water for 10 minutes.
4. Drain the water and run cold water over the eggs to stop them from cooking.
5. Peel the eggs and enjoy!

Nutritional information (per egg): Calories: 72, Protein: 6 grams, Fat: 5 grams, Carbohydrates: 0.5 grams, Cholesterol: 185 milligrams

Tips:

- For easier peeling, add a teaspoon of vinegar or baking soda to the water when you cook the eggs.
- If you like your eggs runny, cook them for 7-8 minutes.
- If you like your eggs hard-boiled, cook them for 10-12 minutes.
- Hard-boiled eggs can be stored in the refrigerator for up to 7 days.

Edamame

COOKING TIME: 5 MINUTES | PREP TIME: 5 MINUTES | TOTAL TIME: 10 MINUTES | SERVING SIZE: 1/2 CUP

Ingredients:

- 1 cup frozen shelled edamame
- 1/2 teaspoon sea salt
- 1/4 teaspoon black pepper
- 1/4 teaspoon garlic powder
- 1/4 teaspoon chili powder (optional)

Directions:

1. In a small saucepan, bring 1 inch of water to a boil.
2. Add the edamame and cook for 3-5 minutes, or until heated through.
3. Drain the edamame and rinse with cold water.
4. In a bowl, toss the edamame with the sea salt, black pepper, garlic powder, and chili powder (if using).
5. Serve immediately.

Nutritional information (per serving): Calories: 120, Protein: 8 grams, Carbohydrates: 11 grams, Fiber: 3 grams, Fat: 3 grams

Tips:

1. For a more flavorful snack, try adding a squeeze of fresh lemon juice or a drizzle of olive oil.
2. You can also roast the edamame in the oven for a crispier texture. Preheat the oven to 400°F (200°C). Spread the edamame on a baking sheet and bake for 10 15 minutes, or until golden brown.
3. Edamame is a good source of protein, fiber, and iron, making it a healthy and satisfying snack for people on a bariatric diet.

Chia Seed Pudding

PREP TIME: 5 MINUTES | COOKING TIME: NONE (OVERNIGHT REFRIGERATION REQUIRED) | TOTAL TIME: 5 MINUTES + OVERNIGHT REFRIGERATION | SERVING SIZE: 1 CUP

Ingredients:

- 1/4 cup chia seeds
- 1 cup unsweetened almond milk or other low-fat milk
- 1/4 cup plain Greek yogurt (non-fat or 2%)
- 1/2 teaspoon vanilla extract
- Optional: 1/4 teaspoon cinnamon, pinch of nutmeg, or a few drops of stevia for sweetness

Directions:

1. In a bowl or jar, combine the chia seeds, almond milk, Greek yogurt, and vanilla extract. Stir well to ensure the chia seeds are evenly distributed.
2. Cover the bowl or jar and refrigerate for at least 4 hours, or preferably overnight. The chia seeds will absorb the liquid and thicken into a pudding-like consistency.
3. In the morning or when ready to enjoy, stir the pudding again. Feel free to add any toppings you like, such as fresh fruit, nuts, seeds, or a drizzle of honey or maple syrup.

Nutritional Information (per serving): Calories: 220, Protein: 10g, Fiber: 6g, Fat: 8g, Carbohydrates: 12g (including 5g of sugar)

Tips:

- For a thicker pudding, use less liquid. For a thinner pudding, use more liquid.
- You can use any type of milk you like, but unsweetened almond milk or coconut milk are good options for a bariatric diet.
- If you don't have Greek yogurt, you can use regular yogurt, but it will be less protein-rich.
- Get creative with your toppings! Try different fruits, nuts, seeds, or spices to find your favorite combinations.
- This pudding can be stored in the refrigerator for up to 3 days.

Turkey Jerky

PREP TIME: 10 MINUTES | MARINATING TIME: 4-8 HOURS, OR OVERNIGHT | COOKING TIME: 4-6 HOURS | TOTAL TIME: 4-14 HOURS | SERVING SIZE: 1

Ingredients:

- 1 pound lean ground turkey
- 1/4 cup low-sodium soy sauce
- 2 tablespoons Worcestershire sauce
- 1 tablespoon brown sugar
- 1 teaspoon garlic powder
- 1/2 teaspoon onion powder
- 1/4 teaspoon black pepper
- 1/4 teaspoon smoked paprika (optional)

Directions:

1. In a large bowl, combine the ground turkey, soy sauce, Worcestershire sauce, brown sugar, garlic powder, onion powder, black pepper, and smoked paprika (if using) Mix well to coat the turkey evenly.
2. Cover the bowl and refrigerate for at least 4 hours, or overnight.
3. Preheat your oven to the lowest setting (usually around 150°F).
4. Line a baking sheet with parchment paper and spread the marinated turkey in a thin layer.
5. Bake for 4-6 hours, or until the jerky is dry and brittle. Be sure to flip the jerky halfway through cooking so it dries evenly.
6. Let the jerky cool completely before storing it in an airtight container.

Nutritional Information: Calories: 70, Protein: 14 grams, Fat: 1 gram, Carbs: 0 grams

Tips:

- You can use a dehydrator instead of an oven to make turkey jerky. If you do, follow the instructions that came with your dehydrator.
- For a thicker jerky, cut the ground turkey into thin strips before marinating.
- If you like your jerky spicy, you can add a pinch of cayenne pepper to the marinade.
- Store turkey jerky in a cool, dry place for up to 2 weeks.

Roasted Chickpeas

PREP TIME: 10 MINUTES | COOK TIME: 40 MINUTES | TOTAL TIME: 50 MINUTES | SERVING SIZE: 1/2 CUP

Ingredients:

- 1 can (15 Oz) chickpeas, drained and rinsed
- 1 tablespoon olive oil
- 1/2 teaspoon dried oregano
- 1/4 teaspoon garlic powder
- 1/4 teaspoon smoked paprika
- Salt and pepper to taste

Directions:

1. Preheat oven to 400°F (200°C).
2. In a large bowl, toss chickpeas with olive oil, oregano, garlic powder, paprika, salt, and pepper.
3. Spread chickpeas on a baking sheet in a single layer.
4. Roast for 40 minutes, or until chickpeas are golden brown and crispy, stirring occasionally.
5. Let cool slightly before serving.

Nutritional Information (per serving): Calories: 150, Fat: 3g, Carbohydrates: 15g, Fiber: 5g, Protein: 8g

Tips:

- For a spicier snack, add a pinch of cayenne pepper.
- If you don't have paprika, you can substitute chili powder.
- Roasted chickpeas can be stored in an airtight container at room temperature for up to 3 days.

Caprese Skewers

COOKING TIME: 10 MINUTES | PREP TIME: 15 MINUTES | TOTAL TIME: 25 MINUTES | SERVING SIZE: 8 SKEWERS

Ingredients:

- 1 pound cherry tomatoes
- 1/2 pound fresh mozzarella cheese balls, cut into bite-sized pieces
- 1/4 cup fresh basil leaves
- 1 tablespoon olive oil
- 1/2 teaspoon balsamic vinegar
- 1/4 teaspoon dried oregano
- Salt and pepper to taste
- 8 bamboo skewers

Directions:

1. Wash the cherry tomatoes and basil leaves.
2. Cut the mozzarella cheese balls into bite-sized pieces.
3. Assemble the skewers by threading a cherry tomato, a mozzarella cheese ball, and a basil leaf onto each skewer.
4. In a small bowl, whisk together the olive oil, balsamic vinegar, oregano, salt, and pepper.
5. Brush the skewers with the dressing.
6. Grill the skewers for 5-10 minutes, or until the tomatoes are slightly softened and the cheese is melted.
7. Serve immediately.

Nutritional information per serving: Calories: 100, Fat: 5g, Carbohydrates: 5g, Protein: 5g, Fiber: 1g

Tips:

- You can use grape tomatoes instead of cherry tomatoes, if desired.
- If you don't have a grill, you can bake the skewers in the oven at 400 degrees F for 10-15 minutes.
- For a vegetarian option, you can omit the mozzarella cheese.
- To make the skewers ahead of time, simply assemble them and store them in the refrigerator for up to 24 hours.

Cucumber and Hummus Bites

PREP TIME: 10 MINUTES | COOKING TIME: 0 MINUTES | TOTAL TIME: 10 MINUTES | SERVING SIZE: 10 BITES

Ingredients:

- 1 medium cucumber, thinly sliced
- 1/2 cup hummus
- 1/4 cup cherry tomatoes, halved
- 1/4 cup crumbled feta cheese
- Fresh dill, for garnish (optional)

Directions:

1. Wash the cucumber and slice it thinly into rounds.
2. Spread hummus on each cucumber slice.
3. Top with a cherry tomato half and a sprinkle of feta cheese.
4. Garnish with fresh dill, if desired.

Nutritional information per serving: Calories: 100, Carbohydrates: 10 grams, Protein: 4 grams, Fat: 5 grams, Fiber: 1 gram

Tips:

- For a variety of flavors, you can use different types of hummus, such as roasted red pepper hummus or black bean hummus.
- You can also add other toppings to your bites, such as olives, chopped bell peppers, or cucumbers.
- If you are on a very restricted diet, you may need to limit the amount of hummus and feta cheese that you use.

Stuffed Mushrooms with Turkey

COOKING TIME: 15 MINUTES | PREP TIME: 10 MINUTES | TOTAL TIME: 25 MINUTES | SERVING SIZE: 12

Ingredients:

- 12 large white button mushrooms
- 4 Oz ground turkey
- 1/2 cup chopped onion
- 1/4 cup chopped bell pepper
- 1 clove garlic, minced
- 1/4 cup low-fat ricotta cheese
- 1/4 cup chopped fresh parsley
- 1/4 teaspoon dried thyme
- Salt and pepper to taste

Directions:

1. Preheat oven to 375°F (190°C).
2. Gently remove the stems from the mushrooms and discard. Scoop out a little of the flesh from the caps to create a larger cavity, being careful not to tear the mushrooms.
3. Chop the reserved mushroom stems and set aside.
4. In a large skillet, cook the ground turkey over medium heat until browned. Drain any excess fat.
5. Add the onion, bell pepper, and garlic to the skillet and cook until softened, about 5 minutes.
1. [Image of Onion, bell pepper, and garlic]
6. Stir in the ricotta cheese, parsley, thyme, salt, and pepper.
7. Add the reserved chopped mushroom stems and cook for an additional minute.
8. Spoon the filling into the mushroom caps.
9. Place the stuffed mushrooms on a baking sheet and bake for 15 minutes, or until the filling is heated through and the mushrooms are tender.

Nutritional Information (per serving): Calories: 70, Carbohydrates: 2g, Fat: 3g, Protein: 7g

Vegetable Spring Rolls

PREP TIME: 15 MINUTES | COOKING TIME: 5 MINUTES | TOTAL TIME: 20 MINUTES | SERVING SIZE: 8 SPRING ROLLS

Ingredients:

- 8 rice paper wrappers
- 1 cup shredded carrots
- 1 cup shredded cucumber
- 1/2 cup shredded red bell pepper
- 1/4 cup shredded green cabbage
- 1/4 cup cooked quinoa (optional for added protein)
- 1/4 cup chopped fresh cilantro
- 1/4 cup chopped fresh mint
- 1/4 cup low-fat dipping sauce (such as peanut sauce, sweet and sour sauce, or a light vinaigrette)

Directions:

1. Prepare the vegetables: Wash and thinly shred the carrots, cucumber, bell pepper, and cabbage. Place them in separate bowls.
2. Cook the quinoa (optional): If using quinoa, rinse it well and cook according to package instructions. Allow it to cool slightly.
3. Assemble the spring rolls: Fill a shallow dish with warm water. Dip a rice paper wrapper in the water for a few seconds, until softened but not soggy. Lay the wrapper flat on a work surface.
4. Place a small handful of each vegetable in the center of the wrapper, along with some quinoa (if using) and herbs.
5. Fold the bottom of the wrapper up over the filling, then fold in the sides. Roll the wrapper tightly from the bottom up, enclosing the filling.
6. Repeat steps 3-5 with the remaining ingredients to make 8 spring rolls.
7. Serve immediately with your favorite low-fat dipping sauce.

Nutritional Information (per Serving): Calories: 150, Protein: 5g, Carbohydrates: 15g (including 3g fiber), fat: 4g

Deviled Eggs with Avocado

COOKING TIME: 10 MINUTES | PREP TIME: 15 MINUTES | TOTAL TIME: 25 MINUTES | SERVING SIZE: 6 HALVES

Ingredients:

- 6 large eggs
- 1/4 avocado, mashed
- 1 tablespoon plain Greek yogurt
- 1 tablespoon low-fat mayonnaise
- 1/2 teaspoon Dijon mustard
- 1/4 teaspoon paprika
- Pinch of salt and pepper

Directions:

1. Hard boil the eggs: Place the eggs in a saucepan and cover with cold water. Bring to a boil, then immediately remove from heat and cover. Let the eggs sit for 10 minutes, then drain and cool under cold running water. Peel the eggs carefully.
2. Cut the eggs in half: Gently slice each egg in half lengthwise. Carefully remove the yolks and place them in a small bowl.
3. Make the filling: Mash the avocado with a fork until smooth. Add the Greek yogurt, mayonnaise, mustard, paprika, salt, and pepper to the egg yolks and mix well until creamy.
4. Fill the eggs: Pipe or spoon the avocado mixture back into the egg white halves. Garnish with a sprinkle of paprika, if desired.

Nutritional Information (per serving): Calories: 130, Protein: 8g, Fat: 7g (2g saturated), Carbohydrates: 1g, Fiber: 1g

Salsa and Guacamole with Veggie Sticks

SALSA

PREP TIME: 10 MINUTES | COOKING TIME: NONE | TOTAL TIME: 10 MINUTES | SERVING SIZE: 1/4 CUP

Nutritional information (per serving): Calories: 25, Fat: 0.5 g, Carbohydrates: 4 g, Fiber: 1 g, Protein: 1 g

Ingredients:

- 1 Roma tomato, seeded and chopped
- 1/2 cucumber, seeded and chopped
- 1/4 red onion, finely chopped
- 1/4 cup chopped cilantro
- 1 tablespoon lime juice
- 1/2 teaspoon chili powder
- 1/4 teaspoon cumin
- Salt and pepper to taste

Directions:

1. Combine all ingredients in a bowl and stir well.
2. Taste and adjust seasonings as needed.

GUACAMOLE

PREP TIME: 10 MINUTES | COOKING TIME: NONE | TOTAL TIME: 10 MINUTES | SERVING SIZE: 1/4 CUP

Nutritional information (per serving): Calories: 80, Fat: 5 g, Carbohydrates: 7 g, Fiber: 3 g, Protein: 2 g

Ingredients:

- 1 ripe avocado, mashed
- 1/4 cup chopped tomato
- 1/4 cup chopped red onion
- 1 tablespoon lime juice
- 1/2 teaspoon chili powder
- 1/4 teaspoon cumin
- Salt and pepper to taste

Directions:

1. Combine all ingredients in a bowl and stir well.
2. Taste and adjust seasonings as needed.

Tips:

- Use a low-fat yogurt or cottage cheese as a base for the guacamole, if desired.
- Add a few chopped black beans to the salsa for extra protein.
- Serve the salsa and guacamole with a variety of whole-grain crackers or pita bread.

Mini Chicken Lettuce Wraps

Ingredients:

- 1 pound ground chicken
- 1/2 cup chopped onion
- 1/4 cup chopped celery
- 1 clove garlic, minced
- 1/2 teaspoon ginger, minced
- 1/4 cup low-sodium soy sauce
- 1 tablespoon rice vinegar
- 1 tablespoon honey
- 1 teaspoon sriracha
- 1 head of romaine lettuce, leaves separated and washed

Directions:

1. In a large skillet, brown the ground chicken over medium heat. Drain the fat.
2. Add the onion, celery, garlic, and ginger to the skillet and cook until softened, about 5 minutes.
3. In a small bowl, whisk together the soy sauce, rice vinegar, honey, and sriracha.
4. Add the sauce to the skillet and cook for an additional minute.
5. To assemble the lettuce wraps, spoon the chicken mixture into the romaine lettuce leaves.

Nutritional information (per serving): Calories: 150, Protein: 15 grams, Carbs: 5 grams, Fat: 5 grams

Tips:

- You can use ground turkey or ground pork instead of ground chicken.
- If you don't have any sriracha, you can use another hot sauce or chili flakes.
- Serve the lettuce wraps with a side of chopped fresh cilantro or chopped peanuts.

Cheese and Turkey Roll-Ups

COOKING TIME: N/A | PREP TIME: 15 MINUTES | TOTAL TIME: 15 MINUTES | SERVING SIZE: 2 ROLL-UPS

Ingredients:

- 2 whole-wheat tortillas (60-70 calories each)
- 4 tablespoons light cream cheese (30 calories per tablespoon)
- 4 slices deli turkey (30 calories per slice)
- 4 spinach leaves
- 2 slices cucumber, thinly sliced
- 1/4 cup shredded reduced-fat cheddar cheese (30 calories per 1/4 cup)
- Freshly ground black pepper, to taste

Directions:

1. Spread 2 tablespoons of light cream cheese onto each tortilla. Leave a 1-inch border around the edges.
2. Top each tortilla with 2 spinach leaves, 2 slices of turkey, and the cucumber slices.
3. Season with black pepper to taste.
4. Tightly roll up each tortilla from the short end.
5. Wrap each roll-up in plastic wrap and refrigerate for at least 30 minutes to allow the flavors to meld and the filling to set.
6. Slice each roll-up into 1-inch pieces and serve chilled.

Nutritional Information (per serving): Calories: 180, Protein: 15g, Carbohydrates: 12g (net 8g), fat: 8g, Fiber: 2g

Tips:

- For added flavor, mix the cream cheese with chopped fresh herbs like dill or chives.
- Substitute turkey with lean ham or roast beef for variety.
- Add other bariatric-friendly vegetables like sliced red bell pepper, shredded carrots, or chopped celery.
- Use low-fat or fat-free cheese for an even lower-fat option.
- Be mindful of portion sizes and consult a registered dietitian for personalized recommendations.

Tuna Cucumber Bites

COOKING TIME: 5 MINUTES | PREP TIME: 10 MINUTES | TOTAL TIME: 15 MINUTES | SERVING SIZE: 12 BITES

Ingredients:

- 1 can (12 Oz) tuna, packed in water, drained and flaked
- 1/2 cup finely chopped celery
- 1/4 cup finely chopped red onion
- 1/4 cup chopped fresh dill
- 1 tablespoon light mayonnaise
- 1 tablespoon Dijon mustard
- 1/2 teaspoon lemon juice
- Salt and pepper to taste
- 12 cucumber slices

Directions:

1. In a medium bowl, combine the tuna, celery, red onion, dill, mayonnaise, Dijon mustard, lemon juice, salt, and pepper. Mix well to combine.
2. Spread about 1 tablespoon of the tuna mixture onto each cucumber slice.
3. Serve immediately or chill for up to 30 minutes before serving.

Nutritional information (per bite): Calories: 50, Protein: 4 grams, Fat: 2 grams, Carbohydrates: 2 grams

Tips:

- For a lower-calorie option, use fat-free mayonnaise or Greek yogurt instead of regular mayonnaise.
- You can also add other chopped vegetables to the tuna mixture, such as bell peppers, carrots, or zucchini.
- If you don't have fresh dill, you can use 1 teaspoon of dried dill weed.
- These bites can be made ahead of time and stored in the refrigerator for up to 24 hours.

Baked Buffalo Cauliflower Bites

PREP TIME: 10 MINUTES | COOK TIME: 25 MINUTES | TOTAL TIME: 35 MINUTES | SERVING SIZE: 1 CUP

Ingredients:

- 1 head cauliflower, cut into bite-sized florets
- 1/4 cup all-purpose flour
- 1/2 teaspoon paprika
- 1/4 teaspoon garlic powder
- 1/4 teaspoon onion powder
- 1/8 teaspoon black pepper
- 1/4 cup unsweetened almond milk
- 1/4 cup hot sauce (such as Frank's Red Hot)
- 1 tablespoon melted light butter
- 1 tablespoon chopped fresh parsley (optional)

Directions:

1. Preheat oven to 400°F (200°C). Line a baking sheet with parchment paper.
2. In a medium bowl, whisk together flour, paprika, garlic powder, onion powder, and black pepper.
3. Gradually add almond milk to the flour mixture, whisking until smooth. The batter should be thin and pourable.
4. Add cauliflower florets to the batter and toss to coat.
5. Spread the coated cauliflower in a single layer on the prepared baking sheet.
6. Bake for 20 minutes, or until the cauliflower is tender and slightly golden brown.
7. In a small bowl, whisk together hot sauce and melted butter.
8. Remove the cauliflower from the oven and brush with the buffalo sauce mixture.
9. Return the cauliflower to the oven and bake for an additional 5 minutes, or until crispy.
10. Garnish with chopped parsley, if desired.

Nutritional Information (per serving): Calories: 150, Fat: 5g, Carbohydrates: 15g, Fiber: 3g, Protein: 8g

Roasted Brussels sprouts

COOKING TIME: 20-25 MINUTES | PREP TIME: 10 MINUTES | TOTAL TIME: 30-35 MINUTES | SERVING SIZE: 1/2 CUP

Ingredients:

- 1 pound Brussels sprouts, trimmed and halved
- 1 tablespoon olive oil
- 1/2 teaspoon salt
- 1/4 teaspoon black pepper
- Optional: 1/4 teaspoon red pepper flakes, 1/4 cup chopped walnuts, 1 tablespoon balsamic vinegar

Directions:

1. Preheat oven to 400 degrees F (200 degrees C).
2. Toss Brussels sprouts with olive oil, salt, and pepper. Spread in a single layer on a baking sheet.
3. Roast for 20-25 minutes, or until tender and browned.
4. Serve immediately.

Nutritional information (per serving): Calories: 50, Carbs: 5 grams, Fiber: 3 grams, Vitamin C: 85% of the RDI, Vitamin K: 130% of the RDI

Tips:

- For added flavor, try adding a teaspoon of garlic powder or dried herbs to the Brussels sprouts before roasting.
- If you like your Brussels sprouts a little crispy, roast them for an additional 5-10 minutes.
- To make a complete meal, add a protein source such as grilled chicken or salmon.
- Brussels sprouts can also be roasted with other vegetables, such as sweet potatoes or carrots.

Cauliflower Mash

COOKING TIME: 15-20 MINUTES | PREP TIME: 5 MINUTES | TOTAL TIME: 20-25 MINUTES | SERVING SIZE: 1/2 CUP (125G)

Ingredients:

- 1 head cauliflower, trimmed and cut into florets
- 1/4 cup unsweetened almond milk (or other low-fat milk)
- 1/4 teaspoon garlic powder
- Salt and pepper to taste
- Fresh herbs (optional, such as parsley, chives, or dill)

Directions:

1. Boil the cauliflower: Place the cauliflower florets in a saucepan and cover with water. Bring to a boil, then reduce heat and simmer for 10-15 minutes, or until tender. Drain and return the cauliflower to the saucepan.
2. Mash the cauliflower: Using a hand mixer or potato masher, mash the cauliflower until smooth and creamy. Add the almond milk and blend until incorporated.
3. Season and flavor: Add the garlic powder, salt, and pepper to taste. Mix well.
4. Garnish and serve: If desired, garnish with fresh herbs for added flavor and nutrients. Serve hot as a side dish with protein and other low-carbohydrate vegetables.

Nutritional Information (per serving): Calories: 50, Carbohydrates: 5g (net carbs), Fat: 0g, Protein: 2g, Fiber: 3g, Vitamin C: 50% DV, Potassium: 10% DV

Zucchini Fritters

PREP TIME: 10 MINUTES | COOK TIME: 10-12 MINUTES | TOTAL TIME: 20-22 MINUTES | SERVING SIZE: 1 FRITTER

Ingredients:

- 1 medium zucchini, grated
- 1/4 cup chopped onion
- 1/4 cup chopped red bell pepper
- 1/4 cup chopped green bell pepper
- 1/4 cup chopped fresh parsley
- 1/4 cup chopped fresh cilantro
- 1/4 cup all-purpose flour (or gluten-free flour blend)
- 1/4 teaspoon baking powder
- 1/4 teaspoon salt
- 1/4 teaspoon black pepper
- 1 egg
- 1 tablespoon olive oil

Directions:

1. In a large bowl, combine the grated zucchini, onion, bell peppers, parsley, cilantro, flour, baking powder, salt, and pepper.
2. In a separate bowl, whisk together the egg and olive oil.
3. Add the egg mixture to the zucchini mixture and stir until well combined.
4. Heat a large skillet over medium heat. Add a thin layer of olive oil to the pan.
5. Using a spoon, drop heaping tablespoons of the zucchini mixture into the pan.
6. Cook the fritters for 3-4 minutes per side, or until golden brown and cooked through.
7. Serve the fritters hot with your favorite dipping sauce, such as yogurt sauce, hummus, or guacamole.

Nutritional Information (per Serving): Calories: 50, Fat: 2g, Carbohydrates: 5g, Fiber: 1g, Protein: 2g

Sautéed Spinach with Garlic

COOKING TIME: 5 MINUTES | PREP TIME: 5 MINUTES | TOTAL TIME: 10 MINUTES | SERVING SIZE: 1 CUP

Ingredients:

- 1 tablespoon olive oil
- 2 cloves garlic, minced
- 10 ounces fresh spinach, washed and stemmed
- Salt and pepper to taste

Directions:

1. Heat olive oil in a large skillet over medium heat.
2. Add garlic and cook for 30 seconds, until fragrant.
3. Add spinach and cook for 3-5 minutes, or until wilted.
4. Season with salt and pepper to taste.
5. Serve immediately.

Nutritional information (per serving): Calories: 41, Carbohydrates: 2 grams, Fiber: 1 gram, Protein: 2 grams, Fat: 2 grams, Vitamin A: 138% of the Daily Value (DV), Vitamin C: 18% of the DV, Vitamin K: 16% of the DV, Iron: 13% of the DV

Tips:

- You can add other vegetables to this dish, such as mushrooms, onions, or bell peppers.
- For a richer flavor, add a sprinkle of Parmesan cheese or a squeeze of lemon juice.
- If you don't have fresh spinach, you can use frozen spinach. Just thaw it in the microwave before adding it to the pan.
- Spinach is a great source of nutrients, including vitamins A, C, and K, iron, and folate. It's also low in calories and carbs, making it a perfect food for a bariatric diet.

Baked Sweet Potato Wedges

COOKING TIME: 25 MINUTES | PREP TIME: 15 MINUTES | TOTAL TIME: 40 MINUTES | SERVING SIZE: 1 WEDGE

Ingredients:

- 1 sweet potato
- 1 tablespoon olive oil
- 1/2 teaspoon sea salt
- 1/4 teaspoon black pepper

Directions:

1. Preheat oven to 400 degrees F (200 degrees C).
2. Wash the sweet potato and cut it into wedges.
3. Toss the sweet potato wedges with olive oil, sea salt, and black pepper.
4. Spread the wedges out on a baking sheet in a single layer.
5. Bake for 25 minutes, or until tender and golden brown.
6. Serve immediately.

Nutritional information: Calories: 100, Fat: 0 grams, Carbohydrates: 25 grams, Fiber: 4 grams, Protein: 2 grams

Tips:

- For a sweeter flavor, try using honey or maple syrup instead of olive oil.
- If you like your wedges crispy, try coating them in a light dusting of cornstarch before baking.
- You can also add other spices to the wedges, such as chili powder, cumin, or paprika.

Quinoa Salad

COOKING TIME: 15 MINUTES | PREP TIME: 10 MINUTES | TOTAL TIME: 25 MINUTES | SERVING SIZE: 1 CUP

Ingredients:

- 1 cup quinoa, rinsed
- 1 cup chopped vegetables (such as bell peppers, cucumbers, carrots, or tomatoes)
- 1/2 cup cooked black beans, rinsed and drained
- 1/4 cup chopped fresh cilantro
- 2 tablespoons olive oil
- 1 tablespoon lemon juice
- 1/2 teaspoon salt
- 1/4 teaspoon black pepper

Directions:

1. In a medium saucepan, combine quinoa and 2 cups of water. Bring to a boil, then reduce heat to low, cover, and simmer for 15 minutes, or until quinoa is cooked and fluffy.
2. While the quinoa is cooking, chop the vegetables and cilantro.
3. In a large bowl, combine the cooked quinoa, vegetables, black beans, and cilantro.
4. In a small bowl, whisk together the olive oil, lemon juice, salt, and pepper. Pour the dressing over the salad and toss to combine.
5. Serve immediately.

Nutritional information (per serving): Calories: 220, Carbohydrates: 35g, Protein: 8g, Fat: 4g, Fiber: 4g

Tips:

- For added protein, you can add grilled chicken, shrimp, or tofu to the salad.
- If you don't have fresh cilantro, you can use 1 teaspoon of dried cilantro.
- To make this salad ahead of time, simply cook the quinoa and prepare the vegetables the day before. Store the salad in an airtight container in the refrigerator for up to 3 days.

Cucumber Avocado Salad

COOKING TIME: NONE | PREP TIME: 10 MINUTES | TOTAL TIME: 10 MINUTES | SERVING SIZE: 1 CUP

Ingredients:

- 1 cucumber, thinly sliced
- 1 avocado, halved, pitted, and sliced
- 1/2 red onion, finely chopped (optional)
- 1/4 cup cherry tomatoes, halved
- 1/4 cup chopped fresh cilantro
- 2 tablespoons fresh lime juice
- 1 tablespoon olive oil
- Salt and pepper to taste

Directions:

1. In a large bowl, combine the sliced cucumber, avocado, red onion (if using), cherry tomatoes, and cilantro.
2. In a separate small bowl, whisk together the lime juice, olive oil, salt, and pepper.
3. Pour the dressing over the salad and toss gently to combine.
4. Serve immediately, chilled.

Nutritional Information (per serving): Calories: 140, Carbohydrates: 6g, Fiber: 3g, Fat: 10g (mostly healthy fats from avocado), Protein: 2g, Vitamin C: 30% Daily Value, Potassium: 10% Daily Value

Tips:

- For a creamier salad, mash some of the avocado with a fork before adding it to the bowl.
- You can add other vegetables like bell peppers, carrots, or radishes to the salad for additional nutrients and flavor.
- For a protein boost, add crumbled cooked chicken or shrimp to the salad.
- This salad is best enjoyed fresh, but you can store any leftovers in an airtight container in the refrigerator for up to 24 hours. However, the avocado may brown slightly.

Broccoli and Cheese Stuffed Peppers

PREP TIME: 10 MINUTES | COOK TIME: 20 MINUTES | TOTAL TIME: 30 MINUTES | SERVING SIZE: 1 PEPPER

Ingredients:

- 2 bell peppers
- 1 cup broccoli florets
- 1/2 cup shredded cheddar cheese
- 1/4 cup chopped onion
- 1 clove garlic, minced
- 1/2 teaspoon Italian seasoning
- 1/4 teaspoon salt
- 1/4 teaspoon black pepper
- 1/4 cup low-fat yogurt

Directions:

1. Preheat oven to 375 degrees F (190 degrees C).
2. Cut the tops off the peppers and remove the seeds and membranes.
3. Blanch the broccoli florets in boiling water for 2 minutes. Drain and set aside.
4. In a bowl, combine the cheddar cheese, onion, garlic, Italian seasoning, salt, and pepper.
5. Add the broccoli florets to the cheese mixture and stir to combine.
6. Spoon the mixture into the hollowed-out peppers.
7. Place the peppers in a baking dish and add 1/4 cup of water to the bottom of the dish.
8. Bake for 20 minutes, or until the peppers are tender and the cheese is melted.
9. Serve with a dollop of low-fat yogurt.

Nutritional information (per serving): Calories: 220, Fat: 10g, Carbohydrates: 20g, Protein: 15g, Fiber: 3g

Tips:

- You can use any type of cheese you like in this recipe.
- If you don't have fresh broccoli, you can use frozen broccoli florets.
- To make this recipe vegan, you can use vegan cheese and yogurt.
- You can also add other vegetables to the filling, such as chopped carrots or zucchini.

Asparagus Wrapped in Turkey Bacon

COOKING TIME: 15-20 MINUTES | PREP TIME: 5 MINUTES | TOTAL TIME: 20-25 MINUTES | SERVING SIZE: 1

Ingredients:

- 6 asparagus spears
- 3 slices turkey bacon
- 1/2 teaspoon olive oil
- Salt and pepper to taste

Directions:

1. Preheat oven to 400 degrees F (200 degrees C).
2. Wash the asparagus and trim off the ends.
3. Cut each turkey bacon slice in half.
4. Wrap each asparagus spear with a half slice of turkey bacon.
1. [Image of Asparagus Wrapped in Turkey Bacon sides]
5. Drizzle the asparagus with olive oil and season with salt and pepper.
6. Place the asparagus on a baking sheet and bake for 15-20 minutes, or until tender and crispy.

Nutritional information (per serving): Calories: 100, Carbohydrates: 5 grams, Protein: 10 grams, Fat: 5 grams

Tips:

- You can use any type of bacon you like, but turkey bacon is a good choice for a bariatric diet because it is lower in fat than regular bacon.
- If you don't have turkey bacon, you can use lean ham or prosciutto.
- You can also grill the asparagus instead of baking it.
- Serve this dish with a low-fat dipping sauce, such as balsamic vinegar or Greek yogurt.

Cabbage Slaw

COOKING TIME: 5 MINUTES | PREP TIME: 10 MINUTES | TOTAL TIME: 15 MINUTES |SERVING SIZE: 1 CUP

Ingredients:

- 1/2 head of green cabbage, thinly sliced
- 1/4 cup red cabbage, thinly sliced (optional)
- 1/4 cup carrots, thinly sliced
- 2 tablespoons apple cider vinegar
- 1 tablespoon Dijon mustard
- 1/2 teaspoon honey
- Salt and pepper to taste

Directions:

1. In a large bowl, combine the cabbage, carrots, and any other desired vegetables.
2. In a small bowl, whisk together the apple cider vinegar, Dijon mustard, and honey.
3. Pour the dressing over the vegetables and toss to coat.
4. Season with salt and pepper to taste.
5. Serve immediately, or refrigerate for up to 2 days.

Nutritional Information (per serving): Calories: 25, Carbohydrates: 4 grams, Fiber: 2 grams, Protein: 1 gram, Fat: 0 grams

Tips:

- You can add other vegetables to this slaw, such as broccoli, cucumber, or bell peppers.
- For a sweeter slaw, use more honey.
- For a spicier slaw, add a pinch of cayenne pepper.
- This slaw can be served as a side dish or topped on grilled chicken or fish.

Grilled Chicken Caesar Salad

COOKING TIME: 10 MINUTES | PREP TIME: 15 MINUTES | TOTAL TIME: 25 MINUTES | SERVING SIZE: 1 LARGE SALAD

Ingredients:

- 4 ounces boneless, skinless chicken breast
- 1 tablespoon olive oil
- 1/2 teaspoon salt
- 1/4 teaspoon black pepper
- 1 head romaine lettuce, chopped
- 1/2 cup cherry tomatoes, halved
- 1/4 cup crumbled Parmesan cheese
- 2 tablespoons Caesar salad dressing (bariatric-friendly)

Directions:

1. Preheat grill to medium heat.
2. In a small bowl, whisk together olive oil, salt, and pepper. Brush the chicken breast with the mixture.
3. Grill the chicken breast for 5-7 minutes per side, or until cooked through.
4. While the chicken is cooking, chop the romaine lettuce and tomatoes.
5. Place the chopped lettuce in a large bowl. Top with the grilled chicken, tomatoes, Parmesan cheese, and Caesar salad dressing.
6. Toss to combine and serve immediately.

Nutritional information (per serving): Calories: 350, Carbohydrates: 7 grams, Fiber: 3 grams, Protein: 30 grams, Fat: 15 grams

Mango and Avocado Salad

COOKING TIME: N/A | PREP TIME: 10 MINUTES | TOTAL TIME: 10 MINUTES | SERVING SIZE: 1 CUP

Ingredients:

- 1 cup romaine lettuce, chopped
- 1/2 ripe mango, diced
- 1/2 ripe avocado, diced
- 1/4 red onion, thinly sliced (optional)
- 1 tablespoon fresh lime juice
- 1 tablespoon olive oil
- Salt and pepper to taste

Directions:

1. Wash and chop the romaine lettuce. Place it in a bowl.
2. Dice the mango and avocado. Add them to the bowl with the lettuce.
3. If using, thinly slice the red onion and add it to the bowl.
4. In a separate bowl, whisk together the lime juice and olive oil. Season with salt and pepper to taste.
5. Drizzle the dressing over the salad and toss to combine.
6. Serve immediately.

Nutritional Information (per serving): Calories: 200 (approximately), Fat: 12g (primarily healthy fats from avocado), Carbohydrates: 15g (mostly from natural sugars in mango), Protein: 2g, Fiber: 4g, Vitamins: A, C, E, K, Minerals: Potassium, magnesium, manganese

Caprese Salad

COOKING TIME: N/A | PREP TIME: 10 MINUTES | TOTAL TIME: 10 MINUTES | SERVING SIZE: 1 CUP

Ingredients:

- 1 medium ripe tomato, sliced
- 4 ounces low-fat mozzarella cheese, sliced or cubed (such as part-skim mozzarella or fresh mozzarella string cheese)
- 1/2 cup baby spinach or arugula
- 1/4 cup chopped fresh basil
- 1 tablespoon balsamic vinegar or olive oil
- Salt and pepper to taste

Directions:

1. Wash and slice the tomato. If using fresh mozzarella string cheese, pull it into bite-sized pieces. If using sliced mozzarella, tear or cut into smaller pieces.
2. Arrange the tomato slices on a plate. Top with the mozzarella cheese and leafy greens.
3. Sprinkle with chopped basil. Drizzle with balsamic vinegar or olive oil.
4. Season with salt and pepper to taste.

Nutritional Information (per serving): Calories: 150, Fat: 5 grams, Carbohydrates: 10 grams, Protein: 8 grams, Fiber: 2 grams

Tips:

- For added protein, sprinkle on some grilled chicken or fish.
- To make it a more substantial meal, add a whole-wheat roll or some quinoa.
- Get creative with the cheese! Use ricotta cheese, cottage cheese, or even goat cheese for a different flavor.
- If you're not on a strict bariatric diet, you can use full-fat mozzarella cheese. Just be mindful of your portion size.

Tuna and White Bean Salad

COOKING TIME: 5 MINUTES (IF USING CANNED TUNA) | PREP TIME: 10 MINUTES | TOTAL TIME: 15 MINUTES | SERVING SIZE: 1 CUP

Ingredients:

- 1 (12-ounce) can tuna, packed in water, drained and flaked
- 1 (15-ounce) can cannellini beans, rinsed and drained
- 1/2 cup chopped cucumber
- 1/2 cup chopped tomato
- 1/4 cup chopped red onion
- 2 tablespoons olive oil
- 2 tablespoons lemon juice
- 1 tablespoon fresh dill, chopped
- 1/2 teaspoon salt
- 1/4 teaspoon black pepper

Directions:

1. In a large bowl, combine the tuna, beans, cucumber, tomato, and red onion.
2. In a small bowl, whisk together the olive oil, lemon juice, dill, salt, and pepper.
3. Pour the dressing over the salad and toss to coat.
4. Serve immediately.

Nutritional information (per serving): Calories: 200, Fat: 5 grams, Carbohydrates: 20 grams, Fiber: 5 grams, Protein: 25 grams

Tips:

- For a heartier salad, add cooked quinoa or brown rice.
- If you don't have fresh dill, you can use 1 teaspoon dried dill.
- You can also use other types of beans, such as chickpeas or kidney beans.
- If you prefer, you can grill the tuna instead of using canned tuna.

Cobb Salad

COOKING TIME: 10 MINUTES | PREP TIME: 15 MINUTES | TOTAL TIME: 25 MINUTES | SERVING SIZE: 1

Ingredients:

- 4 ounces grilled chicken breast, sliced
- 2 ounces lean ham, diced
- 1/2 cup crumbled blue cheese
- 1/2 avocado, sliced
- 1 hard-boiled egg, sliced
- 1/2 cup chopped tomatoes
- 1/4 cup chopped red onion
- 1/4 cup chopped cucumber
- 2 tablespoons crumbled bacon
- 2 tablespoons olive oil
- 1 tablespoon lemon juice
- 1/2 teaspoon dried oregano
- 1/4 teaspoon salt
- 1/4 teaspoon black pepper

Directions:

1. Preheat a grill or grill pan to medium heat. Grill the chicken breast until cooked through, about 10 minutes. Let cool slightly and then slice.
2. In a large bowl, combine the chicken, ham, blue cheese, avocado, egg, tomatoes, red onion, and cucumber.
3. In a small bowl, whisk together the olive oil, lemon juice, oregano, salt, and pepper.
4. Pour the dressing over the salad and toss to coat.
5. Sprinkle with bacon and serve immediately.

Nutritional Information: Calories: 300, Protein: 30 grams, Fat: 10 grams, Carbohydrates: 15 grams, Fiber: 5 grams

Roasted Beet and Goat Cheese Salad

COOKING TIME: 20 MINUTES | PREP TIME: 15 MINUTES | TOTAL TIME: 35 MINUTES | SERVING SIZE: 1

Ingredients:

- 2 medium beets, trimmed and chopped into wedges
- 1 tablespoon olive oil
- 1/2 teaspoon dried thyme
- Salt and pepper to taste
- 4 cups mixed greens
- 4 ounces goat cheese, crumbled
- 1/4 cup chopped walnuts
- 2 tablespoons balsamic vinegar
- 1 tablespoon olive oil

Directions:

1. Preheat oven to 400°F (200°C).
2. Toss beets with olive oil, thyme, salt, and pepper. Spread on a baking sheet in a single layer.
3. Roast for 20 minutes, or until tender and slightly browned.
4. While beets are roasting, prepare the salad. Place mixed greens in a large bowl.
5. Once beets are cooked, add them to the salad bowl along with goat cheese, walnuts, balsamic vinegar, and olive oil. Toss gently to combine.
6. Serve immediately.

Nutritional information (per serving): Calories: 300, Carbohydrates: 25 grams, Fat: 15 grams, Protein: 10 grams, Fiber: 5 grams

Tips:

- For a heartier salad, add grilled chicken or shrimp.
- If you don't have balsamic vinegar, you can use red wine vinegar or lemon juice.
- To make this salad ahead of time, simply roast the beets and store them in an airtight container in the refrigerator for up to 3 days. Assemble the salad just before serving.

Shrimp and Avocado Salad

PREP TIME: 10 MINUTES | COOK TIME: 5 MINUTES | TOTAL TIME: 15 MINUTES | SERVING SIZE: 1 CUP

Ingredients:

- 1 pound shrimp, peeled and deveined
- 1 avocado, diced
- 1 cucumber, diced
- 1 tomato, diced
- 1/2 red onion, diced
- 1/4 cup chopped cilantro
- 2 tablespoons lime juice
- 1 tablespoon olive oil
- Salt and pepper to taste

Directions:

1. Bring a pot of water to a boil. Add the shrimp and cook for 3-5 minutes, or until pink and cooked through. Drain and cool slightly.
2. In a large bowl, combine the shrimp, avocado, cucumber, tomato, red onion, and cilantro.
3. In a small bowl, whisk together the lime juice and olive oil. Season with salt and pepper to taste.
4. Pour the dressing over the salad and toss to combine. Serve immediately.

Nutritional information: Calories: 250, Protein: 20 grams, Fat: 15 grams, Carbohydrates: 5 grams

Tips:

- You can use grilled or boiled shrimp for this recipe.
- If you are on a very strict bariatric diet, you may need to omit the avocado or use a smaller amount.
- This salad is a great source of protein, fiber, and healthy fats. It is also very refreshing and flavorful.

Kale and Berry Salad

COOKING TIME: 5 MINUTES | PREP TIME: 10 MINUTES | TOTAL TIME: 15 MINUTES | SERVING SIZE: 1

Ingredients:

- 1 cup kale, chopped
- 1/2 cup mixed berries (such as blueberries, raspberries, and strawberries)
- 1/4 cup cooked quinoa (optional)
- 1/4 cup crumbled feta cheese (optional)
- 1/4 cup chopped walnuts or pecans
- 2 tablespoons olive oil
- 1 tablespoon lemon juice
- 1/2 teaspoon Dijon mustard
- Salt and pepper to taste

Directions:

1. Wash and chop the kale. Place it in a large bowl.
2. Add the berries, quinoa (if using), feta cheese (if using), and nuts to the bowl.
3. In a small bowl, whisk together the olive oil, lemon juice, Dijon mustard, salt, and pepper.
4. Pour the dressing over the salad and toss to coat.
5. Serve immediately.

Nutritional Information (per serving): Calories: 250, Fat: 5 grams, Carbohydrates: 35 grams, Fiber: 5 grams, Protein: 5 grams, Vitamin A: 120% DV, Vitamin C: 100% DV, Potassium: 20% DV

Tips:

- For a more flavorful salad, marinate the berries in the dressing for 30 minutes before adding them to the salad.
- If you don't have quinoa, you can use another cooked grain, such as brown rice or barley.
- You can also add other vegetables to the salad, such as chopped cucumber, shredded carrots, or bell peppers.
- If you're not on a bariatric diet, you can increase the serving size or add additional toppings, such as grilled chicken or shrimp.

Egg Salad Lettuce Wraps

COOKING TIME: 10 MINUTES | PREP TIME: 15 MINUTES | TOTAL TIME: 25 MINUTES | SERVING SIZE: 2

Ingredients:

- 2 romaine lettuce leaves
- 2 hard-boiled eggs, chopped
- 1/4 cup chopped celery
- 1/4 cup chopped red onion
- 1 tablespoon plain Greek yogurt
- 1 teaspoon Dijon mustard
- 1/2 teaspoon lemon juice
- Salt and pepper to taste

Directions:

1. Bring a pot of water to a boil. Carefully add the eggs and cook for 10 minutes. Drain the water and let the eggs cool slightly, then peel and chop them.
2. In a medium bowl, combine the chopped eggs, celery, red onion, Greek yogurt, Dijon mustard, lemon juice, salt, and pepper. Stir until well combined.
3. Wash and dry the romaine lettuce leaves. Fill each leaf with a generous scoop of the egg salad mixture.

Nutritional information (per wrap): Calories: 150, Fat: 8g, Carbs: 5g, Fiber: 2g, Protein: 12g

Tips:

- For a creamier egg salad, use more Greek yogurt.
- Add other chopped vegetables to the salad, such as cucumbers or bell peppers.
- If you don't have romaine lettuce, you can use any other type of lettuce or leafy green.
- Serve the wraps with a side of sliced fruit or yogurt for a complete meal.

Mexican Cauliflower Rice Salad

COOKING TIME: N/A | PREP TIME: 15 MINUTES | TOTAL TIME: 15 MINUTES | SERVING SIZE: 1 CUP

Ingredients:

- 2 cups cauliflower rice (freshly riced or frozen)
- 1/2 cup black beans, rinsed and drained
- 1/2 cup corn kernels (fresh or frozen)
- 1/4 cup red bell pepper, diced
- 1/4 cup red onion, diced
- 1/4 cup cilantro, chopped
- 2 tablespoons lime juice
- 1 tablespoon olive oil
- 1/2 teaspoon cumin
- 1/4 teaspoon chili powder
- Pinch of salt and pepper

Directions:

1. Combine the cauliflower rice, black beans, corn, bell pepper, red onion, and cilantro in a large bowl.
2. Whisk together the lime juice, olive oil, cumin, chili powder, salt, and pepper in a small bowl.
3. Pour the dressing over the salad ingredients and toss to combine.
4. Chill for at least 15 minutes before serving, allowing the flavors to meld.

Nutritional Information (per serving): Calories: 150, Carbohydrates: 10g (net), Protein: 5g, Fat: 5g, Fiber: 3g

Tips:

- For a spicier salad, add a seeded and finely chopped jalapeño pepper to the ingredients.
- If you prefer a warmer salad, sauté the corn kernels in a little olive oil before adding them to the bowl.
- This salad can be stored in an airtight container in the refrigerator for up to 3 days.
- Feel free to customize this recipe by adding other vegetables or herbs, such as chopped tomatoes, avocado, or jicama.

LIQUID RECIPES

Protein-Packed Smoothie

COOKING TIME: N/A | PREP TIME: 5 MINUTES | TOTAL TIME: 5 MINUTES | SERVING SIZE: 1 (16 OZ) SMOOTHIE

Ingredients:

- 1 scoop unflavored protein powder (whey, pea, or plant-based)
- 1 cup unsweetened almond milk or other low-fat milk alternative
- 1/2 cup frozen berries (mixed berries, blueberries, raspberries, etc.)
- 1/2 banana
- 1/4 cup spinach or other leafy greens (optional)
- 1/4 teaspoon ground cinnamon
- 1/4 cup ice

Directions:

1. Add all ingredients to a blender and blend until smooth and creamy.
2. Pour into a glass and enjoy immediately.

Nutritional Information (per Serving): Calories: 350-400 (depending on ingredients), Protein: 25-30 grams, Carbohydrates: 20-25 grams, Fat: 5-10 grams, Fiber: 5-10 grams, Vitamins and Minerals: Varies depending on ingredients used

Tips:

- Use frozen fruits for a thicker and colder smoothie.
- Add a scoop of nut butter for extra protein and healthy fats.
- Use unsweetened Greek yogurt for an even creamier and more protein-rich smoothie.
- Adjust the sweetness to your preference using stevia or other natural sweeteners.
- Feel free to experiment with different fruits, vegetables, and spices to find your perfect combination.

Green Protein Shake

COOKING TIME: N/A | PREP TIME: 5 MINUTES | TOTAL TIME: 5 MINUTES | SERVING SIZE: 16 OUNCES

Ingredients:

- 1 cup leafy greens (spinach, kale, collard greens)
- 1/2 cup frozen berries (mixed berries, blueberries, raspberries)
- 1/2 cup banana (optional)
- 1/2 cup unsweetened almond milk (or preferred unsweetened milk)
- 1/2 cup non-fat Greek yogurt (or lactose-free alternative)
- 1 scoop unflavored protein powder (bariatric-friendly)
- 1/4 tsp. vanilla extract (optional)
- Ice cubes (optional)

Directions:

1. Wash and chop your leafy greens if not already pre-washed.
2. Combine all ingredients in a blender and blend until smooth and creamy.
3. Add ice cubes for a thicker and colder consistency, if desired.
4. Enjoy immediately!

Nutritional Information (per serving): Calories: 250-300 (depending on chosen ingredients),Protein: 20 25 grams (depending on chosen protein powder), Carbohydrates: 15 20 grams (depending on chosen fruits and vegetables), Fat: 5-10 grams (depending on chosen yogurt and milk), Fiber: 2-4 grams (depending on chosen fruits and vegetables), Vitamins and Minerals: Varies depending on ingredients, but typically rich in Vitamins A, C, K, folate, and potassium.

Creamy Avocado Soup

PREP TIME: 10 MINUTES | COOK TIME: 15 MINUTES | TOTAL TIME: 25 MINUTES | SERVING SIZE: 1 CUP

Ingredients:

- 1 ripe avocado, pitted and chopped
- 1 cup low-sodium chicken broth
- 1/2 cup low-fat plain yogurt
- 1/4 cup chopped red onion
- 1 clove garlic, minced
- 1 tablespoon fresh lime juice
- 1/2 teaspoon dried cilantro
- Salt and pepper to taste

Instructions:

1. In a large saucepan, combine the chicken broth, red onion, garlic, and cilantro. Bring to a boil, then reduce heat and simmer for 5 minutes.
2. Add the avocado and yogurt to the saucepan and blend until smooth using an immersion blender or blender.
3. Stir in the lime juice, salt, and pepper to taste.
4. Serve hot or cold.

Nutritional information per serving: Calories: 200, Fat: 14g, Carbohydrates: 5g, Fiber: 4g, Protein: 2g, Vitamin A: 20% DV, Vitamin C: 30% DV, Potassium: 20% DV

Tips:

- For a thicker soup, use less chicken broth.
- For a thinner soup, use more chicken broth.
- You can also add other vegetables to the soup, such as chopped carrots or celery.
- If you don't have cilantro, you can use parsley instead.
- This soup can be stored in the refrigerator for up to 3 days.

Berry Protein Popsicles

COOKING TIME: 0 MINUTES | PREP TIME: 10 MINUTES | TOTAL TIME: 10 MINUTES | SERVING SIZE: 1 POPSICLE

Ingredients:

* 1/2 cup plain Greek yogurt
* 1/2 cup unsweetened almond milk
* 1/4 cup mixed berries (fresh or frozen)
* 1 scoop vanilla protein powder
* 1/4 teaspoon honey (optional)

Directions:

1. In a blender, combine the Greek yogurt, almond milk, berries, protein powder, and honey (if using). Blend until smooth.
2. Pour the mixture into Popsicle molds.
3. Freeze for at least 4 hours, or until solid.

Nutritional information (per Popsicle): Calories: 100, Protein: 10 grams, Carbohydrates: 15 grams, Fat: 1 gram, Fiber: 2 grams

Tips:

* You can use any type of protein powder you like. Just make sure it's a bariatric-friendly brand.
* If you don't have Popsicle molds, you can use small paper cups or ice cube trays.
* Get creative with the flavors! Try adding other fruits, such as mango, pineapple, or peaches. You can also add a teaspoon of chia seeds or flaxseeds for extra nutrients.
* These popsicles are best enjoyed within a week of being made.

Chocolate Peanut Butter Protein Shake

COOKING TIME: 2 MINUTES | PREP TIME: 5 MINUTES | TOTAL TIME: 7 MINUTES | SERVING SIZE: 1

Ingredients:

- 1 scoop chocolate protein powder
- 1/2 cup unsweetened almond milk
- 1/4 cup unsweetened natural peanut butter
- 1/2 frozen banana
- 1/4 cup ice cubes
- 1/4 teaspoon vanilla extract
- Pinch of cinnamon (optional)

Directions:

1. Combine all ingredients in a blender and blend until smooth and creamy.
2. Pour into a glass and enjoy!

Nutritional information: Calories: 340, Carbohydrates: 25 grams, Protein: 25 grams, Fat: 10 grams, Fiber: 4 grams, Sugar: 10 grams

Tips:

- For a thicker shake, use less almond milk.
- For a thinner shake, use more almond milk.
- You can add other fruits or vegetables to this shake, such as spinach, kale, or berries.
- If you don't have protein powder, you can use Greek yogurt instead.
- This shake is also a great breakfast or snack option.

Tomato Basil Soup

COOKING TIME: 15 MINUTES | PREP TIME: 10 MINUTES | TOTAL TIME: 25 MINUTES | SERVING SIZE: 1 CUP

Ingredients:

- 1 tablespoon olive oil
- 1 onion, chopped
- 2 cloves garlic, minced
- 1 (28-ounce) can crushed tomatoes
- 4 cups low-sodium chicken broth
- 1 tablespoon chopped fresh basil
- 1/2 teaspoon dried oregano
- Salt and pepper to taste
- 1/4 cup low-fat Greek yogurt (optional)

Directions:

1. Heat olive oil in a large saucepan over medium heat. Add onion and cook until softened, about 5 minutes.
2. Add garlic and cook for 1 minute more.
3. Stir in crushed tomatoes, chicken broth, basil, oregano, salt, and pepper. Bring to a boil, then reduce heat and simmer for 15 minutes.
4. Puree the soup with an immersion blender or in batches in a blender until smooth.
5. Return the soup to the saucepan and heat through.
6. Serve hot, garnished with a dollop of low-fat Greek yogurt, if desired.

Nutritional information per serving: Calories: 120, Fat: 2g, Carbohydrates: 14g, Protein: 10g, Fiber: 3g, Vitamin A: 15% DV, Vitamin C: 30% DV, Potassium: 10% DV

Mocha Protein Frappe

COOKING TIME: N/A | PREP TIME: 5 MINUTES | TOTAL TIME: 5 MINUTES | SERVING SIZE: 1 FRAPPE

Ingredients:

- 1 scoop unflavored protein powder (whey or plant-based)
- 1 cup unsweetened almond milk (or other bariatric-friendly milk substitute)
- 1/2 cup strong coffee, chilled
- 1/4 cup plain Greek yogurt (optional, for added creaminess)
- 1 tablespoon unsweetened cocoa powder
- 1/4 teaspoon vanilla extract
- 1/4 cup ice cubes
- Stevia or your preferred sweetener (to taste)

Directions:

1. Combine all ingredients in a blender and blend until smooth and frothy.
2. Adjust the sweetness to your preference with stevia or your preferred sweetener.
3. Pour into a glass and enjoy immediately.

Nutritional Information (per serving): Calories: 250-300 (depending on ingredients used), Protein: 20-25 grams, Carbohydrates: 15-20 grams, Fat: 5-10 grams, Fiber: 2-3 grams

Tips:

- For a thicker and creamier frappe, use frozen coffee cubes instead of regular ice cubes.
- You can add a pinch of cinnamon or nutmeg for extra flavor.
- If you don't have plain Greek yogurt, you can use a dollop of whipped cream (bariatric-friendly option) for added protein and creaminess.
- Use unsweetened almond milk or another bariatric-friendly milk substitute to keep the calorie and sugar content low.
- This recipe is easily customizable. Feel free to add other bariatric-friendly ingredients like berries, spinach, or nut butter for additional nutrients and flavor.

Spicy Veggie Broth

COOKING TIME: 20 MINUTES | PREP TIME: 10 MINUTES | TOTAL TIME: 30 MINUTES | SERVING SIZE: 1 CUP

Ingredients:

- 1 tablespoon olive oil
- 1 onion, chopped
- 2 carrots, chopped
- 2 celery stalks, chopped
- 1 clove garlic, minced
- 4 cups vegetable broth
- 1 teaspoon dried thyme
- 1/2 teaspoon dried oregano
- 1/4 teaspoon red pepper flakes (optional)
- Salt and pepper to taste
- Chopped fresh parsley, for garnish (optional)

Directions:

1. Heat olive oil in a large pot or Dutch oven over medium heat. Add onion, carrots, and celery, and cook until softened, about 5 minutes.
2. Add garlic and cook for 1 minute more.
3. Pour in vegetable broth, thyme, oregano, and red pepper flakes (if using). Bring to a boil, then reduce heat and simmer for 15 minutes.
4. Season with salt and pepper to taste. Garnish with chopped fresh parsley, if desired.

Nutritional information per serving: Calories: 30, Carbs: 3 grams, Fiber: 1 gram, Protein: 1 gram, Fat: 0 grams, Sugar: 2 grams, Sodium. 400mg

Tips:

- You can use any type of vegetable you like in this broth. Some other good options include bell peppers, mushrooms, and zucchini.
- If you don't have vegetable broth, you can use water instead. Just be sure to add a little more salt to taste.
- This broth can be stored in the refrigerator for up to 3 days. Reheat gently before serving.

Cucumber Mint Cooler

COOKING TIME: 0 MINUTES | PREP TIME: 5 MINUTES | TOTAL TIME: 5 MINUTES | SERVING SIZE: 1 CUP

Ingredients:

- 1 cup chopped cucumber
- 1/2 cup fresh mint leaves
- 1/4 cup lime juice
- 1/4 cup water
- 1/4 teaspoon stevia, or to taste

Directions:

1. Combine all ingredients in a blender and blend until smooth.
2. Taste and add more stevia, if desired.
3. Serve immediately.

Nutritional information (per serving): Calories: 25, Carbohydrates: 5 grams, Sugar: 4 grams, Fiber: 1 gram, Vitamin C: 14% Daily Value, Potassium: 4% Daily Value

Tips:

- You can use any type of sweetener you like, such as honey, agave nectar, or monk fruit sweetener.
- If you don't have fresh mint, you can use 1 teaspoon of dried mint.
- For a thicker cooler, add 1/2 cup of ice to the blender with the other ingredients.
- This recipe is also great for making ahead of time. Simply store the cooler in the refrigerator for up to 24 hours.

Creamy Chicken Broth

COOKING TIME: 20 MINUTES | PREP TIME: 10 MINUTES | TOTAL TIME: 30 MINUTES | SERVING SIZE: 1 CUP

Ingredients:

- 1 tablespoon olive oil
- 1 onion, chopped
- 2 carrots, chopped
- 2 celery stalks, chopped
- 4 cups chicken broth
- 1 boneless, skinless chicken breast, cooked and shredded
- 1/2 cup nonfat plain Greek yogurt
- 1/4 teaspoon dried thyme
- Salt and pepper to taste

Directions:

1. Heat olive oil in a large saucepan over medium heat. Add onion, carrots, and celery, and cook until softened, about 5 minutes.
2. Add chicken broth and bring to a boil. Reduce heat to simmer and cook for 10 minutes.
3. Add cooked chicken, yogurt, thyme, salt, and pepper. Stir to combine and heat through.
4. Serve immediately.

Nutritional information per serving: Calories: 50, Fat: 1g, Carbohydrates: 5g, Protein: 8g

Tips:

- You can use cooked chicken from a rotisserie chicken to save time.
- If you don't have Greek yogurt, you can use cottage cheese or unsweetened almond milk.
- Add other vegetables to the broth, such as chopped broccoli or mushrooms.
- For a thicker broth, use an immersion blender to puree some of the vegetables before adding the chicken and yogurt.

Pumpkin Spice Protein Smoothie

PREP TIME: 5 MINUTES | COOKING TIME: 0 MINUTES | TOTAL TIME: 5 MINUTES | SERVINGS: 1

Ingredients:

- 1 scoop vanilla protein powder
- 1/2 cup pumpkin puree
- 1/2 cup unsweetened almond milk
- 1/4 cup ice
- 1/2 teaspoon pumpkin spice
- 1/4 teaspoon cinnamon
- Pinch of nutmeg

Directions:

1. Blend all ingredients together in a blender until smooth.
2. Pour into a glass and enjoy!

Nutritional information: Calories: 250, Protein: 25 grams, Carbs: 20 grams, Fat: 5 grams, Fiber: 3 grams, Sugar: 5 grams

Tips:

- Use frozen pumpkin puree for a thicker smoothie.
- Add more protein powder for a boost of protein.
- Use your favorite type of milk or yogurt.
- Add a splash of coffee for a caffeine kick.

Chilled Berry Soup

PREP TIME: 10 MINUTES | COOKING TIME: 15 MINUTES | TOTAL TIME: 25 MINUTES | SERVING SIZE: 1 CUP

Ingredients:

- 1 cup mixed berries (such as strawberries, blueberries, raspberries, and blackberries)
- 1/2 cup water
- 1/4 cup plain Greek yogurt
- 1 tablespoon honey
- 1/2 teaspoon vanilla extract
- Pinch of ground cinnamon

Dircctions:

1. In a small saucepan, combine the berries and watcr. Bring to a boil, then reduce heat and simmer for 10 minutes.
2. Remove from heat and let cool slightly.
3. In a blender, combine the cooled berries, yogurt, honey, vanilla extract, and cinnamon. Blend until smooth.
4. Refrigerate for at least 1 hour before serving.

Nutritional information per serving: Calories: 50, Carbohydrates: 10 grams, Fiber: 2 grams, Protein: 1 gram, Fat: 0 grams

Tips:

- You can use any type of berries you like.
- If you don't have plain Greek yogurt, you can use low-fat or fat-free yogurt.
- If you don't have honcy, you can usc another sweetener, such as stevia or agave nectar.
- You can add a few ice cubes to the soup when you blend it for a thicker consistency.
- This soup is also delicious topped with a dollop of whipped cream or a sprinkle of chopped nuts.

Vanilla Chai Protein Latte

COOKING TIME: 3 MINUTES | PREP TIME: 5 MINUTES | TOTAL TIME: 8 MINUTES | SERVING SIZE: 12 OZ

Ingredients:

- 1/2 cup unsweetened chai tea concentrate (or 1 tea bag steeped in 1/2 cup boiling water for 5 minutes)
- 1 scoop unflavored protein powder (whey or plant-based)
- 1/2 cup unsweetened almond milk (or other low-fat milk)
- 1/4 teaspoon vanilla extract
- Ice cubes (optional)
- Sugar-free sweetener (optional, to taste)

Directions:

1. If using chai tea concentrate, simply measure out 1/2 cup. If using a tea bag, steep it in 1/2 cup boiling water for 5 minutes, then remove the bag and let the tea cool slightly.
2. Add the chai tea concentrate, protein powder, almond milk, and vanilla extract to a blender or shaker cup.
3. Blend or shake until smooth and frothy. If using ice, add it to the blender/shaker cup before blending.
4. Taste and add sugar-free sweetener if desired.
5. Pour into a glass and enjoy!

Nutritional Information per serving: Calories: 150, Protein: 20g, Carbs: 15g, Fat: 5g

Tips:

- You can use any type of unsweetened milk you like, such as soy milk, oat milk, or even water.
- If you don't have chai tea concentrate, you can make your own by simmering chai spices (such as cinnamon, ginger, cardamom, and cloves) in water with honey or sugar-free sweetener.
- For a thicker latte, use less milk. For a thinner latte, use more milk.
- Get creative with toppings! Try adding a sprinkle of cinnamon, nutmeg, or even a dollop of whipped cream (made with sugar-free whipped cream topping).

Ginger Turmeric Elixir

COOKING TIME: 5 MINUTES | PREP TIME: 5 MINUTES | TOTAL TIME: 10 MINUTES | SERVING SIZE: 1 CUP (240 ML)

Ingredients:

- 1 inch fresh ginger, peeled and roughly chopped
- 1/2 inch fresh turmeric, peeled and roughly chopped (or 1 teaspoon ground turmeric)
- 1 cup water
- 1/2 lemon, juiced (optional)
- Honey or stevia to taste (optional)

Directions:

1. Combine ginger, turmeric, and water in a saucepan. Bring to a boil, then reduce heat and simmer for 5 minutes.
2. Strain the mixture through a fine-mesh sieve into a cup.
3. Stir in lemon juice and honey or stevia, if using.
4. Enjoy warm or chilled.

Nutritional Information (per serving): Calories: 25, Carbohydrates: 5g, Sugar: 2g, Fat: 0g, Protein: 0g, Fiber: 1g, Vitamin C: 10% Daily Value, Manganese: 10% Daily Value, Potassium: 5% Daily Value

Tips:

- For a thicker elixir, simmer for an additional 5 minutes until the liquid reduces slightly.
- You can also add other spices like cinnamon, cardamom, or black pepper for additional flavor and nutritional benefits.
- If you don't have fresh ginger or turmeric, you can use 1 teaspoon of ground ginger and 1/2 teaspoon of ground turmeric instead.
- Feel free to adjust the amount of lemon juice and sweetener to your taste.

Creamy Spinach and Artichoke Soup

PREP TIME: 10 MINUTES | COOK TIME: 20 MINUTES | TOTAL TIME: 30 MINUTES | SERVING SIZE: 1 CUP

Ingredients:

- 1 tablespoon olive oil
- 1 onion, chopped
- 2 cloves garlic, minced
- 4 cups chicken broth
- 1 (14.5-ounce) can artichoke hearts, drained and chopped
- 10 ounces frozen spinach
- 1/2 cup low-fat milk
- 1/4 cup sour cream
- 1/4 teaspoon salt
- 1/4 teaspoon black pepper

Directions:

1. Heat olive oil in a large pot over medium heat. Add onion and garlic, and cook until softened, about 5 minutes.
2. Add chicken broth, artichoke hearts, and spinach to the pot. Bring to a boil, then reduce heat and simmer for 10 minutes.
3. In a blender, puree the soup until smooth. Return the soup to the pot and stir in milk, sour cream, salt, and pepper.
4. Heat through, but do not boil. Serve immediately.

Nutritional information: Calories: 150, Fat: 5 grams, Protein: 10 grams, Carbohydrates: 15 grams, Fiber: 5 grams

Tips:

- For a thicker soup, use less milk.
- For a thinner soup, use more milk.
- You can also add other vegetables to this soup, such as carrots, celery, or zucchini.
- If you don't have sour cream, you can use plain Greek yogurt instead.

146 |Bariatric Diet Cookbook

DESSERTS

Protein-Packed Pudding

PREP TIME: 5 MINUTES | COOKING TIME: 15 MINUTES | TOTAL TIME: 20 MINUTES | SERVING SIZE: 1/2 CUP

Ingredients:

- 1 scoop protein powder
- 1/2 cup milk (dairy or non-dairy)
- 1/4 cup Greek yogurt
- 1/4 cup unsweetened applesauce
- 1/4 teaspoon vanilla extract
- 1/4 teaspoon cinnamon

Directions:

1. In a small saucepan, whisk together the protein powder, milk, yogurt, applesauce, vanilla extract, and cinnamon.
2. Cook over medium heat until the mixture thickens and comes to a boil, about 5 minutes.
3. Remove from heat and let cool slightly.
4. Pour into two small dishes or ramekins and refrigerate for at least 2 hours, or until set.

Nutritional information: Calories: 150, Protein: 20 grams, Carbohydrates: 15 grams, Fat: 5 grams

Tips:

- You can use any type of protein powder that you like. Whey protein powder is a good choice for this recipe, but you can also use casein or plant-based protein powder.
- If you don't have applesauce, you can use another type of fruit puree, such as pumpkin puree or mashed banana.
- You can add other toppings to your pudding, such as chopped nuts, seeds, or fresh fruit.

Chia Seed Pudding

PREP TIME: 5 MINUTES | COOKING TIME: 0 MINUTES | TOTAL TIME: 5 MINUTES | SERVING SIZE: 1 CUP

Ingredients:

- 1/4 cup chia seeds
- 1 cup unsweetened almond milk
- 1/2 teaspoon vanilla extract
- 1/4 teaspoon cinnamon
- Optional: sweetener, fruit, nuts, or seeds*

Directions:

1. In a bowl or jar, combine the chia seeds, almond milk, vanilla extract, and cinnamon. Stir well to combine.
2. Let the mixture sit for at least 5 minutes, or until the chia seeds have thickened.
3. Refrigerate for at least 2 hours, or overnight.
4. Serve with your favorite toppings.

Nutritional information per serving: Calories: 230, Fat: 7g, Carbohydrates: 11g, Fiber: 10g, Protein: 6g

Tips:

- *For a thinner pudding, use 1 1/2 cups of almond milk.
- *For a thicker pudding, use 1/2 cup of almond milk.
- *You can use any type of milk you like, but unsweetened almond milk is a good choice for people on a bariatric diet.
- *If you want your pudding to be sweeter, you can add a sweetener of your choice.
- *Top your pudding with your favorite fruits, nuts, or seeds. Some good options include berries, bananas, mangos, almonds, walnuts, and chia seeds.

Baked Apple with Cinnamon

COOKING TIME: 25-30 MINUTES | PREP TIME: 10 MINUTES | TOTAL TIME: 35-40 MINUTES | SERVING SIZE: 1 APPLE

Ingredients:

- 1 medium apple (such as Granny Smith, Gala, or Honey crisp)
- 1/2 teaspoon ground cinnamon
- 1/4 teaspoon ground ginger (optional)
- 1/4 teaspoon lemon juice
- 1 tablespoon chopped walnuts or pecans (optional)
- 1/2 teaspoon honey or maple syrup (optional, for added sweetness)

Directions:

1. Preheat oven to 375°F (190°C).
2. Wash and dry the apple. Core the apple, leaving the bottom intact to create a cup-like shape.
3. In a small bowl, combine cinnamon, ginger (if using), and lemon juice. Brush the inside of the apple with the mixture.
4. Place the apple in a baking dish, cut-side facing up. If desired, sprinkle with chopped nuts and drizzle with honey or maple syrup.
5. Bake for 25-30 minutes, or until the apple is tender and slightly softened.
6. Let the apple cool slightly before enjoying.

Nutritional Information (per serving): Calories: 70-80, Carbohydrates: 15-20 grams, Fiber: 4-5 grams, Sugar: 8-10 grams, Fat: 0-1 gram, Protein: 0-1 gram

Tips:

- For a sweeter filling, add a teaspoon of chopped raisins or dried cranberries to the apple before baking.
- If you don't have fresh ginger, you can substitute 1/8 teaspoon of ground ginger.
- To make this recipe dairy-free, use vegan-friendly honey or maple syrup.
- Serve the baked apple warm or chilled, topped with a dollop of plain Greek yogurt or unsweetened applesauce for an extra protein boost.

Frozen Yogurt Bites

Prep time: 10 minutes

Cooking time: 15 minutes

Total time: 25 minutes

Serving size: 12 bites

Ingredients:

- 1 cup plain Greek yogurt
- 1/4 cup fruit puree (such as mango, strawberry, or blueberry)
- 1/4 teaspoon honey
- 1/4 teaspoon vanilla extract
- Mini muffin tin

Directions:

1. In a bowl, combine the Greek yogurt, fruit puree, honey, and vanilla extract.
2. Pour the mixture into the mini muffin tin, filling each well about 3/4 full.
3. Freeze for at least 15 minutes, or until firm.
4. Enjoy!

Nutritional information: Calories: 50 per bite, Protein: 5 grams per bite, Carbohydrates: 6 grams per bite, Fat: 1 gram per bite

Tips:

- You can use any type of fruit puree that you like.
- If you don't have honey, you can use another sweetener, such as stevia or monk fruit extract.
- You can also add other toppings to your yogurt bites, such as chopped nuts, granola, or mini chocolate chips.

Avocado Chocolate Mousse

COOKING TIME: 5 MINUTES | PREP TIME: 10 MINUTES | TOTAL TIME: 15 MINUTES | SERVING SIZE: 1/2 CUP

Ingredients:

- 1 ripe avocado, pitted and peeled
- 1/4 cup unsweetened cocoa powder
- 2 tablespoons honey or maple syrup
- 1/4 cup almond milk
- 1/4 teaspoon vanilla extract
- Pinch of sea salt

Instructions:

1. Add all ingredients to a blender or food processor.
2. Blend until smooth and creamy, scraping down the sides as needed.
3. Divide the mousse into two small bowls or ramekins.
4. Refrigerate for at least 30 minutes before serving.

Nutritional information (per serving): Calories: 210, Fat: 18g, Carbohydrates: 10g, Fiber: 5g, Protein: 4g, Sugar: 3g

Tips:

- For a richer flavor, use dark chocolate cocoa powder.
- You can also add a scoop of your favorite protein powder to boost the protein content.
- If the mousse is too thick, add a little more almond milk.
- If the mousse is too thin, chill it for longer or add a tablespoon of chia seeds.
- Top your mousse with a sprinkle of chopped nuts, berries, or a drizzle of chocolate sauce.

Sugar-Free Gelatin Cups

COOKING TIME: 10 MINUTES | PREP TIME: 15 MINUTES | TOTAL TIME: 25 MINUTES | SERVING SIZE: 1 CUP

Ingredients:

- 1 packet sugar-free gelatin (any flavor)
- 1 cup unsweetened fruit juice (such as grape, cranberry, or pineapple)
- 1/2 cup boiling water
- 1/4 cup cold water
- 1/4 teaspoon stevia or other sugar-free sweetener

Directions:

1. In a small bowl, whisk together the gelatin and boiling water until the gelatin is dissolved.
2. Stir in the cold water and fruit juice.
3. Add the sweetener to taste.
4. Pour the mixture into individual serving cups or molds.
5. Refrigerate for at least 4 hours, or until set.

Nutritional information (per serving): Calories: 50, Carbohydrates: 8 grams, Fiber: 2 grams, Protein: 4 grams, Fat: 0 grams

Tips:

- For a fun twist, try using different flavors of gelatin and fruit juice.
- You can also add in fresh or frozen fruit for extra flavor and nutrients.
- If you don't have stevia, you can use another sugar-free sweetener, such as sucralose or erythritol.
- These gelatin cups can be stored in the refrigerator for up to 3 days.

Berry Parfait

COOKING TIME: 0 MINUTES | PREP TIME: 10 MINUTES | TOTAL TIME: 10 MINUTES | SERVING SIZE: 1 PARFAIT

Ingredients:

- 1/2 cup plain Greek yogurt
- 1/2 cup fresh berries (such as blueberries, raspberries, or strawberries)
- 1/4 cup granola
- 1/4 teaspoon vanilla extract

Directions:

1. In a small bowl, layer the Greek yogurt, berries, and granola.
2. Drizzle with vanilla extract.
3. Serve immediately.

Nutritional information (per serving): Calories: 250, Protein: 20 grams, Carbohydrates: 25 grams, Fiber: 5 grams, Fat: 5 grams

Tips:

- For a thicker parfait, use frozen berries.
- If you don't have granola, you can use chopped nuts or seeds.
- You can also add a drizzle of honey or maple syrup to the parfait.
- This parfait is a great way to get your daily dose of fruits and yogurt.
- It's also a good source of protein and fiber, which can help you feel full and satisfied.

Coconut Flour Pancakes

COOKING TIME: 10-12 MINUTES | PREP TIME: 5 MINUTES | TOTAL TIME: 15-17 MINUTES | SERVING SIZE: 1 PANCAKE

Ingredients:

- 1/4 cup coconut flour
- 1/2 teaspoon baking powder
- 1/4 teaspoon baking soda
- 1/4 teaspoon salt
- 1 egg
- 1/2 cup unsweetened almond milk
- 1 tablespoon melted coconut oil
- 1/2 teaspoon vanilla extract
- Optional toppings: fresh fruit, berries, whipped cream, sugar-free syrup

Directions:

1. In a medium bowl, whisk together the coconut flour, baking powder, baking soda, and salt.
2. In a separate bowl, whisk together the egg, almond milk, coconut oil, and vanilla extract.
3. Pour the wet ingredients into the dry ingredients and whisk until just combined. Do not over mix.
4. Heat a lightly greased griddle or frying pan over medium heat.
5. Pour about 1/4 cup of batter per pancake onto the griddle.
6. Cook for 2-3 minutes per side, or until golden brown and cooked through.
7. Serve immediately with your desired toppings.

Nutritional Information (per pancake): Calories: 150, Carbohydrates: 5g (net), Fiber: 3g, Protein: 12g, Fat: 8g

Tips:

- For a thicker pancake, add 1-2 tablespoons of chia seeds or ground flaxseed to the batter.
- If the batter is too thick, add a little more almond milk. If it's too thin, add a little more coconut flour.
- You can also make these pancakes in a waffle iron.
- Store leftover pancakes in an airtight container in the refrigerator for up to 3 days.

Peanut Butter Protein Balls

COOKING TIME: 10 MINUTES | PREP TIME: 15 MINUTES | TOTAL TIME: 25 MINUTES | SERVING SIZE: 10 BALLS

Ingredients:

- 1 cup rolled oats
- 1/2 cup peanut butter
- 1/4 cup honey
- 1/4 cup mini chocolate chips
- 1 scoop vanilla protein powder

Directions:

1. In a large bowl, combine the rolled oats, peanut butter, honey, chocolate chips, and protein powder.
2. Mix well until the ingredients are well combined and a dough forms.
3. Roll the dough into 10 balls.
4. Place the balls on a baking sheet lined with parchment paper.
5. Refrigerate for at least 30 minutes, or until firm.
6. Enjoy!

Nutritional information per ball: Calories: 190, Fat: 8 grams, Carbohydrates: 18 grams, Protein: 8 grams, Fiber: 2 grams

Tips:

- You can use any type of nut butter you like, such as almond butter or cashew butter.
- If you don't have mini chocolate chips, you can use chopped nuts or dried fruit.
- You can also make these balls ahead of time and store them in the freezer for up to two weeks.

Baked Peach with Cinnamon

COOKING TIME: 15-20 MINUTES | PREP TIME: 10 MINUTES | TOTAL TIME: 25-30 MINUTES | SERVING SIZE: 1 PEACH HALF

Ingredients:

- 2 ripe peaches, halved and pitted
- 1/2 teaspoon ground cinnamon
- 1/4 cup unsweetened almond milk
- 1/4 teaspoon vanilla extract (optional)
- 1/8 teaspoon ground nutmeg (optional)

Directions:

1. Preheat oven to 375°F (190°C).
2. Place the peach halves, cut-side up, in a baking dish. Sprinkle each half with cinnamon.
3. In a small bowl, whisk together the almond milk, vanilla extract (if using), and nutmeg (if using). Pour the mixture evenly over the peaches.
4. Bake for 15-20 minutes, or until the peaches are softened and lightly browned.
5. Let cool slightly before serving.

Nutritional Information (per serving): Calories: 70, Carbohydrates: 15g, Protein: 1g, Fat: 0g, Fiber: 2g, Sugar: 10g

Tips:

- For a sweeter treat, you can drizzle the peaches with a small amount of honey or maple syrup after baking.
- If you don't have almond milk, you can use water or unsweetened applesauce instead.
- For a thicker sauce, you can mix 1 teaspoon of cornstarch with 1 tablespoon of water before adding it to the milk mixture.
- This recipe can be easily doubled or tripled to serve more people.

SWEET TREATS

Dark Chocolate-Covered Almonds

PREP TIME: 10 MINUTES | COOK TIME: 5 MINUTES | TOTAL TIME: 15 MINUTES | SERVING SIZE: 1/4 CUP

Ingredients:

- 1/2 cup raw almonds
- 1/4 cup dark chocolate chips (60% cacao or higher)
- 1/4 teaspoon coconut oil

Directions:

1. Spread the almonds out on a baking sheet in a single layer.
2. Bake at 350 degrees Fahrenheit for 5 minutes, or until lightly toasted.
3. Melt the chocolate chips and coconut oil in a double boiler or in the microwave in 30-second intervals, stirring until smooth.
4. Let the chocolate cool slightly.
5. Dip the almonds in the chocolate, using a fork or spoon to coat them evenly.
6. Place the coated almonds on a baking sheet lined with parchment paper.
7. Refrigerate for at least 30 minutes, or until the chocolate is hardened.

Nutritional Information: Calories: 150, Fat: 10 grams, Carbohydrates: 8 grams, Protein: 4 grams, Fiber: 2 grams

Tips:

- You can use any type of nuts or seeds that you like in this recipe.
- If you don't have coconut oil, you can use vegetable oil or butter.
- For a fun twist, try adding a sprinkle of sea salt or crushed peppermint to the chocolate before it hardens.

Sugar-Free Popsicles

PREP TIME: 10 MINUTES | COOKING TIME: 15 MINUTES (FREEZING TIME NOT INCLUDED) | TOTAL TIME: 25 MINUTES (PLUS FREEZING TIME) | SERVING SIZE: 1

Ingredients:

- 1 cup unsweetened Greek yogurt
- 1/2 cup chopped fresh fruit (such as berries, mango, or pineapple)
- 1/4 cup water
- 1/4 teaspoon vanilla extract

Directions:

1. In a blender, combine the yogurt, fruit, water, and vanilla extract. Blend until smooth.
2. Pour the mixture into Popsicle molds.
3. Freeze for at least 2 hours, or until solid.
4. Enjoy!

Nutritional Information (per Popsicle): Calories: 50, Fat: 0g, Carbohydrates: 10g, Protein: 2g, Sugar: 5g

Tips:

- You can use any type of fruit you like.
- If the mixture is too thick, add a little more water.
- If the mixture is too thin, add a little more yogurt.
- You can also add other flavorings, such as mint extract or almond extract.
- For a fun twist, try layering different flavors of fruit in the Popsicle molds.

Cottage Cheese with Berries

COOKING TIME: 0 MINUTES | PREP TIME: 5 MINUTES | TOTAL TIME: 5 MINUTES | SERVING SIZE: 1/2 CUP

Ingredients:

- 1/2 cup low-fat cottage cheese
- 1/4 cup berries (such as blueberries, raspberries, or strawberries)
- 1 teaspoon honey or maple syrup (optional)
- 1/4 teaspoon vanilla extract (optional)

Directions:

1. In a small bowl, combine the cottage cheese and berries.
2. If desired, add the honey or maple syrup and vanilla extract.
3. Stir well and enjoy immediately.

Nutritional information (per serving): Calories: 150, Protein: 15g, Carbohydrates: 10g, Fat: 2g, Fiber: 2g, Sugar: 5g

Tips:

- For a thicker treat, use Greek yogurt instead of cottage cheese.
- You can also add other toppings, such as chopped nuts, seeds, or granola.
- If you don't have fresh berries, you can use frozen berries. Just thaw them slightly before adding them to the cottage cheese.

Almond Flour Cookies

PREP TIME: 10 MINUTES | COOK TIME: 10-12 MINUTES | TOTAL TIME: 22 MINUTES | SERVING SIZE: 1 COOKIE

Ingredients:

- 1/2 cup almond flour
- 1/4 cup coconut flour
- 1/4 teaspoon baking soda
- 1/4 teaspoon salt
- 1/4 cup unsalted butter, softened
- 1/4 cup honey
- 1/2 teaspoon vanilla extract
- 1/4 cup chopped nuts (optional

Directions:

1. Preheat oven to 350°F (175°C). Line a baking sheet with parchment paper.
2. In a medium bowl, whisk together almond flour, coconut flour, baking soda, and salt.
3. In a separate bowl, cream together butter and honey until light and fluffy. Beat in vanilla extract.
4. Add the wet ingredients to the dry ingredients and mix until just combined. Fold in chopped nuts, if using.
5. Drop tablespoons of dough onto the prepared baking sheet, leaving about 1 inch of space between cookies.
6. Bake for 10-12 minutes, or until edges are golden brown.
7. Let cookies cool on the baking sheet for a few minutes before transferring to a wire rack to cool completely.

Nutritional Information per Serving: Calories: 120, Fat: 8g, Carbohydrates: 8g (net carbs 3g), Fiber: 3g, Protein: 3g, Sugar: 3g

Tips:

- For a chewier cookie, bake for less time. For a crispier cookie, bake for a minute or two longer.
- You can substitute the chopped nuts with your favorite sugar-free chocolate chips or dried fruit.
- Store cookies in an airtight container at room temperature for up to 3 days.
- Freeze cookies for longer storage.

Frozen Banana Bites

PREP TIME: 10 MINUTES | COOKING TIME: 20 MINUTES (FREEZING TIME) | TOTAL TIME: 30 MINUTES | SERVING SIZE: 10 BITES

Ingredients:

- 2 ripe bananas
- 1/4 cup Greek yogurt
- 1/4 cup dark chocolate chips
- 1 tablespoon chopped nuts (optional)

Directions:

1. Peel and slice the bananas into 1-inch thick rounds.
2. Spread the Greek yogurt evenly over the banana slices.
3. Sprinkle the chocolate chips and nuts (if using) over the yogurt.
4. Place the banana slices on a baking sheet lined with parchment paper.
5. Freeze for at least 20 minutes, or until firm.

Nutritional Information: Calories: 50 per bite, Protein: 1 gram per bite, Carbohydrates: 11 grams per bite, Fat: 0 grams per bite, Fiber: 1 gram per bite

Tips:

- You can use any type of yogurt you like, but Greek yogurt is a good source of protein.
- If you don't have dark chocolate chips, you can use semisweet chocolate chips or even chopped nuts.
- For a more decadent treat, you can dip the frozen banana bites in melted chocolate.
- If you are following a strict bariatric diet, be sure to check the nutritional information of all of the ingredients you use.

Baked Berry Crisp

PREP TIME: 15 MINUTES | COOK TIME: 25 MINUTES | TOTAL TIME: 40 MINUTES | SERVING SIZE: 1/2 CUP

Ingredients:

- **Crisp Topping:**
- 1/4 cup oat bran
- 1/4 cup almond flour
- 1/4 cup chopped pecans or walnuts
- 1/4 teaspoon ground cinnamon
- 1/4 teaspoon nutmeg
- 1 tablespoon cold unsalted butter, cubed
- 1-2 tablespoons stevia or monk fruit sweetener (to taste)
- **Berry Filling:**
- 1 cup mixed berries (fresh or frozen)
- 1/4 cup plain Greek yogurt (2%)
- 1 tablespoon lemon juice
- 1 teaspoon cornstarch

Instructions:

1. Preheat oven to 375°F (190°C). Lightly grease a small baking dish (6x6 inches or similar).
2. Crisp Topping: Combine oat bran, almond flour, nuts, cinnamon, and nutmeg in a bowl. Using a pastry cutter or your fingers, work in the butter until it forms coarse crumbs. Stir in sweetener until evenly distributed.
3. Berry Filling: In a separate bowl, mix berries, Greek yogurt, lemon juice, and cornstarch. Toss gently to coat the berries.
4. Pour the berry mixture into the prepared baking dish. Sprinkle the crisp topping evenly over the berries.
5. Bake for 25-30 minutes, or until the topping is golden brown and the filling is bubbly.
6. Let cool slightly before serving. Enjoy warm or at room temperature.

Nutritional Information per Serving: Calories: 180, Protein: 8g, Carbohydrates: 25g (7g fiber), fat: 5g, Sugar: 5g (from natural sources and sweetener)

Mini Cheesecake Bites

PREP TIME: 15 MINUTES | COOKING TIME: 15 MINUTES | TOTAL TIME: 30 MINUTES | SERVING SIZE: 12 BITES

Ingredients:

- 1/2 cup graham cracker crumbs
- 1 tablespoon melted butter
- 1/4 cup light cream cheese
- 1/4 cup unsweetened applesauce
- 1/4 cup plain Greek yogurt
- 1 egg
- 1/2 teaspoon vanilla extract
- 1/4 teaspoon sugar
- 12 fresh strawberries

Directions:

1. Preheat oven to 350 degrees F (175 degrees C).
2. In a medium bowl, combine the graham cracker crumbs and melted butter. Press the mixture into the bottom of a 12-cup muffin tin.
3. In a large bowl, beat together the cream cheese, applesauce, yogurt, egg, vanilla extract, and sugar until smooth.
4. Divide the cheesecake filling evenly among the muffin cups.
5. Bake for 15 minutes, or until the filling is set.
6. Let the cheesecakes cool in the muffin tin for 10 minutes, then transfer them to a wire rack to cool completely.
7. Top each cheesecake with a fresh strawberry.

Nutritional information: Calories: 50 per bite, Fat: 2 grams per bite, Carbohydrates: 7 grams per bite, Protein: 2 grams per bite

Tips:

- You can use any type of fruit you like for the topping.
- If you don't have a muffin tin, you can use a mini cheesecake pan.
- These cheesecakes can be stored in the refrigerator for up to 3 days.

Strawberry Shortcake

PREP TIME: 10 MINUTES | COOK TIME: 15 MINUTES | TOTAL TIME: 25 MINUTES | SERVING SIZE: 1 SHORTCAKE

Ingredients:

- 1/2 cup whole wheat pastry flour
- 1/4 teaspoon baking powder
- 1/4 teaspoon salt
- 1 tablespoon cold unsalted butter, cut into cubes
- 1/4 cup nonfat Greek yogurt
- 1 tablespoon honey
- 1/4 cup chopped fresh strawberries

Directions:

1. Preheat oven to 375 degrees F (190 degrees C). Lightly grease a baking sheet.
2. In a medium bowl, whisk together flour, baking powder, and salt.
3. Using a pastry cutter or your fingers, cut the butter into the flour mixture until it resembles coarse crumbs.
4. Stir in the yogurt and honey until a dough forms.
5. Knead the dough on a lightly floured surface a few times until just smooth.
6. Pat the dough out into a circle about 1/2 inch thick.
7. Cut out 2 rounds of dough with a 2-inch biscuit cutter.
8. Place the dough rounds on the prepared baking sheet.
9. Bake for 15 minutes, or until golden brown.
10. Let the shortcakes cool slightly before serving.
11. Top each shortcake with 1/4 cup chopped strawberries.

Nutritional information: Calories: 250, Carbohydrates: 30 grams, Protein: 8 grams, Fat: 5 grams, Fiber: 3 grams

Pumpkin Spice Protein Shake

PREP TIME: 5 MINUTES | COOKING TIME: 0 MINUTES | TOTAL TIME: 5 MINUTES | SERVING SIZE: 1 POPSICLE

Ingredients:

- 1 scoop vanilla protein powder
- 1/2 cup unsweetened almond milk
- 1/4 cup canned pumpkin puree
- 1/2 teaspoon pumpkin spice
- 1/4 teaspoon ground cinnamon
- 1/8 teaspoon ground nutmeg
- 1/4 cup ice cubes

Directions:

1. Combine all ingredients in a blender and blend until smooth.
2. Pour into Popsicle molds and freeze for at least 2 hours.

Nutritional information: Calories: 100, Protein: 15g, Carbohydrates: 10g, Fat: 2g, Fiber: 2g

Tips:

- For a thicker shake, use less almond milk or add a thickening agent like xanthan gum.
- For a sweeter shake, add a few drops of stevia or monk fruit extract.
- You can also add other fall spices to the shake, such as ginger or cloves.

Homemade Protein Ice Cream

PREP TIME: 10 MINUTES | COOK TIME: 5 MINUTES | TOTAL TIME: 15 MINUTES | SERVINGS: 2

Ingredients:

- 1 scoop vanilla protein powder (1/2 cup)
- 1/2 cup unsweetened almond milk
- 1/4 cup frozen berries (such as strawberries, blueberries, or raspberries)
- 1/4 teaspoon vanilla extract
- 1/4 cup ice cubes

Directions:

1. In a blender, combine protein powder, almond milk, berries, vanilla extract, and ice cubes.
2. Blend until smooth and creamy.
3. Serve immediately.

Nutritional Information: Calories: 200, Fat: 5 grams, Carbohydrates: 15 grams, Protein: 20 grams

Tips:

- For a thicker ice cream, use less almond milk or freeze the mixture for 30 minutes before blending.
- You can use any type of protein powder you like.
- Feel free to add in other flavors, such as chocolate chips, nuts, or peanut butter.
- If you don't have a blender, you can use a food processor.

RECIPES FOR CHRISTMAS AND NEW YEAR CELEBRATIONS

Herb-Roasted Turkey Breast

COOKING TIME: 1 HOUR 30 MINUTES | PREP TIME: 15 MINUTES | TOTAL TIME: 1 HOUR 45 MINUTES | SERVING SIZE: 1

Ingredients:

- 4-ounce boneless, skinless turkey breast
- 1 tablespoon olive oil
- 1/2 teaspoon dried thyme
- 1/2 teaspoon dried rosemary
- 1/4 teaspoon salt
- 1/4 teaspoon black pepper
- 1/4 cup chicken broth

Directions:

1. Preheat oven to 350°F (175°C).
2. Pat the turkey breast dry with paper towels.
3. In a small bowl, combine olive oil, thyme, rosemary, salt, and pepper. Rub the mixture all over the turkey breast.
4. Place the turkey breast in a baking dish and pour the chicken broth around it.
5. Cover the dish with foil and bake for 1 hour.
6. Remove the foil and bake for an additional 30 minutes, or until the turkey breast is cooked through and golden brown.
7. Let the turkey breast rest for 5 minutes before slicing and serving.

Nutritional information per serving: Calories: 170, Fat: 5 grams, Carbohydrates: 2 grams, Protein: 30 grams

Cauliflower Mash

COOKING TIME: 15 MINUTES | PREP TIME: 10 MINUTES | TOTAL TIME: 25 MINUTES | SERVING SIZE: 1 CUP

Ingredients:

- 1 head cauliflower, cut into florets
- 1/4 cup unsweetened almond milk
- 2 tablespoons low-fat Greek yogurt
- 1/2 teaspoon garlic powder
- 1/4 teaspoon salt
- 1/4 teaspoon black pepper

Directions:

1. Preheat oven to 400°F (200°C).
2. Place cauliflower florets on a baking sheet and roast for 15 minutes, or until tender.
3. Transfer roasted cauliflower to a blender or food processor.
4. Add almond milk, yogurt, garlic powder, salt, and pepper.
5. Blend until smooth and creamy.
6. Serve immediately.

Nutritional information per serving: Calories: 50, Carbohydrates: 5g, Fiber: 3g, Protein: 2g, Fat: 0g

Tips:

- For a richer flavor, add a tablespoon of grated Parmesan cheese to the blender.
- You can also roast the cauliflower with a drizzle of olive oil for added flavor.
- If you don't have almond milk, you can use water or broth.
- Leftovers can be stored in an airtight container in the refrigerator for up to 3 days.

Here are some additional details that you may find helpful:

Green Bean Almondine

COOKING TIME: 10-15 MINUTES | PREP TIME: 5 MINUTES | TOTAL TIME: 20 MINUTES | SERVING SIZE: 1/2 CUP

Ingredients:

- 1 pound fresh green beans, trimmed and halved
- 1 tablespoon olive oil
- 1/4 cup slivered almonds
- 1/4 cup low-sodium chicken broth
- 1/4 teaspoon lemon juice
- Salt and freshly ground black pepper to taste

Directions:

1. In a large pot, bring a pot of salted water to a boil. Add the green beans and cook for 3-4 minutes, or until tender-crisp. Drain and rinse with cold water to stop the cooking process.
2. Heat the olive oil in a large skillet over medium heat. Add the almonds and cook, stirring frequently, until lightly toasted and golden brown. Remove from the heat and set aside.
3. Add the chicken broth to the skillet and bring to a simmer. Stir in the lemon juice, salt, and pepper.
4. Add the green beans back to the skillet and toss to coat in the sauce. Heat through for another minute or two.
5. Garnish with the toasted almonds and serve immediately.

Nutritional Information (per serving): Calories: 70, Fat: 3g (less than 1g saturated), Carbohydrates: 10g (4g fiber), Protein: 3g, Sodium: 130mg

Tips:

- For a protein boost, add a grilled chicken breast or shrimp to the dish.
- To make it even lighter, use vegetable broth instead of chicken broth.
- If you're feeling adventurous, try adding a pinch of cayenne pepper for a kick.
- Leftovers can be stored in an airtight container in the refrigerator for up to 3 days.

Bariatric-friendly Gravy

PREP TIME: 5 MINUTES | COOK TIME: 10 MINUTES | TOTAL TIME: 15 MINUTES | SERVING SIZE: 1/4 CUP

Ingredients:

- 1 tablespoon cornstarch
- 1 cup unsweetened low-sodium chicken broth
- 1/2 teaspoon dried thyme
- 1/4 teaspoon black pepper
- Dash of garlic powder

Directions:

1. In a small bowl, whisk together the cornstarch and 2 tablespoons of the chicken broth until smooth.
2. In a medium saucepan, whisk together the remaining chicken broth, thyme, pepper, and garlic powder. Bring to a boil over medium heat.
3. Slowly whisk in the cornstarch mixture and cook until the gravy thickens, about 1 minute.
4. Reduce heat to low and simmer for 5 minutes, stirring occasionally.
5. Serve immediately over your favorite bariatric-friendly protein, such as grilled chicken or fish.

Nutritional information per serving: Calories: 25, Fat: 0g, Carbohydrates: 4g, Protein: 1g, Sodium: 120mg

Tips:

- For a richer flavor, you can add 1 tablespoon of low-fat sour cream or Greek yogurt to the gravy.
- You can also use this recipe to make gravy for mashed potatoes, vegetables, or rice.
- If you don't have cornstarch, you can use arrowroot powder or xanthan gum instead.
- Be sure to use low-sodium chicken broth to keep the sodium content of the gravy down.

Spinach and Feta Stuffed Mushrooms

PREP TIME: 15 MINUTES | COOKING TIME: 15 MINUTES | TOTAL TIME: 30 MINUTES | SERVING SIZE: 6

Ingredients:

- 6 large portobello mushrooms
- 1 tablespoon olive oil
- 1/2 small onion, chopped
- 2 cloves garlic, minced
- 10 ounces fresh spinach, chopped
- 1/4 cup crumbled feta cheese
- 1/4 teaspoon dried oregano
- Salt and pepper to taste

Directions:

1. Preheat oven to 375 degrees F (190 degrees C).
2. Clean the mushrooms by wiping them with a damp paper towel. Remove the stems and gently scrape out the gills with a spoon.
3. Heat olive oil in a large skillet over medium heat. Add onion and garlic and cook until softened, about 5 minutes.
4. Add spinach and cook until wilted, about 2 minutes.
5. Remove from heat and stir in feta cheese, oregano, salt, and pepper.
6. Spoon the spinach and feta mixture into the portobello mushroom caps.
7. Bake in the preheated oven for 15 minutes, or until the mushrooms are tender and the filling is heated through.
8. Serve immediately.

Nutritional information per serving: Calories: 150, Protein: 8 grams, Carbohydrates: 10 grams, Fat: 8 grams, Fiber: 2 grams

Tips:

- You can use other types of cheese in this recipe, such as ricotta cheese or mozzarella cheese.
- To make this recipe vegan, use vegan feta cheese and omit the oregano.
- You can also add other ingredients to the filling, such as chopped sun-dried tomatoes or cooked crumbled sausage.

Baked Salmon with Lemon-Dill Sauce

COOKING TIME: 15 MINUTES | PREP TIME: 10 MINUTES | TOTAL TIME: 25 MINUTES | SERVING SIZE: 1 FILLET (4 OUNCES)

Ingredients:

- 1 salmon fillet (4 ounces)
- 1/4 teaspoon salt
- 1/4 teaspoon black pepper
- 1 tablespoon olive oil
- 1/4 cup lemon juice
- 1/4 cup chopped fresh dill
- 1 tablespoon chopped fresh parsley

Directions:

1. Preheat oven to 400 degrees F (200 degrees C).
2. Season the salmon fillet with salt and pepper.
3. Place the salmon in a baking dish and drizzle with olive oil.
4. In a small bowl, whisk together the lemon juice, dill, and parsley.
5. Pour the lemon-dill sauce over the salmon.
6. Bake for 15 minutes, or until the salmon is cooked through.
7. Serve immediately.

Nutritional information per serving: Calories: 250, Protein: 30 grams, Fat: 10 grams, Carbohydrates: 5 grams

Tips:

- You can also use skinless, boneless salmon fillets for this recipe.
- If you don't have fresh dill, you can use 1 teaspoon of dried dill.
- To make this recipe even more flavorful, you can marinate the salmon in the lemon-dill sauce for 30 minutes before baking.
- Serve this dish with roasted vegetables or a side salad.

Brussels sprouts with Bacon

PREP TIME: 10 MINUTES | COOK TIME: 20 MINUTES | TOTAL TIME: 30 MINUTES | SERVING SIZE: 1 CUP

Ingredients:

- 1 pound Brussels sprouts, trimmed and halved
- 4 slices bacon, chopped
- 1/2 onion, chopped
- 1 tablespoon olive oil
- 1/4 teaspoon salt
- 1/4 teaspoon black pepper

Directions:

1. Preheat oven to 400 degrees F (200 degrees C).
2. In a large bowl, toss Brussels sprouts with olive oil, salt, and pepper.
3. Spread the Brussels sprouts on a baking sheet in a single layer.
4. Roast for 20 minutes, or until tender and slightly browned.
5. While the Brussels sprouts are roasting, cook the bacon in a skillet over medium heat until crispy.
6. Drain the bacon on paper towels.
7. Add the onion to the skillet and cook until softened, about 5 minutes.
8. Add the cooked bacon and onion to the roasted Brussels sprouts.
9. Serve immediately.

Nutritional information (per serving): Calories: 180, Fat: 10 grams, Protein: 15 grams, Carbohydrates: 10 grams, Fiber: 5 grams

Tips:

- You can also add other vegetables to this dish, such as chopped carrots or bell peppers.
- If you don't have bacon, you can use turkey bacon or ham.
- To make this dish vegan, omit the bacon and use olive oil instead of bacon fat.

Crustless Pumpkin Pie

COOKING TIME: 50-55 MINUTES | PREP TIME: 10 MINUTES | TOTAL TIME: 60-65 MINUTES | SERVING SIZE: 1/8 PIE

Ingredients:

- 1 can (15 Oz) pumpkin puree (unsweetened)
- 1 cup unsweetened almond milk
- 4 large eggs, separated
- 1/4 cup Splenda or other sugar substitute (adjust to taste)
- 1 tsp. ground cinnamon
- 1/2 tsp. ground ginger
- 1/4 tsp. ground nutmeg
- 1/8 tsp. ground cloves
- Pinch of salt

Directions:

1. Preheat oven to 350°F (175°C). Grease a 9-inch pie dish with cooking spray.
2. In a large bowl, whisk together pumpkin puree, almond milk, egg yolks, Splenda, spices, and salt until smooth.
3. In a separate bowl, whisk egg whites until stiff peaks form. Gently fold egg whites into the pumpkin mixture until just combined.
4. Pour the batter into the prepared pie dish. Bake for 50-55 minutes, or until the center is set and a toothpick inserted comes out clean.
5. Let the pie cool completely on a wire rack before serving. Chill for at least 2 hours for a firmer texture.

Nutritional Information (per serving): Calories: 150-175 (depending on ingredients used), Protein: 8-10 grams, Carbs: 15-20 grams, Fat: 5-7 grams, Fiber: 2-3 grams

Tips:

- For a richer flavor, add 1 tablespoon of sugar-free vanilla extract to the batter.
- Top your pie with a dollop of sugar-free whipped cream or Greek yogurt for an extra treat.
- Store leftover pie in the refrigerator for up to 3 days.

Cucumber and Tomato Salad

COOKING TIME: 0 MINUTES | PREP TIME: 10 MINUTES | TOTAL TIME: 10 MINUTES | SERVING SIZE: 1 CUP

Ingredients:

- 1 cucumber, thinly sliced
- 1 tomato, thinly sliced
- 1/4 red onion, thinly sliced
- 1/4 cup chopped fresh parsley
- 2 tablespoons olive oil
- 1 tablespoon lemon juice
- 1/2 teaspoon dried oregano
- Salt and pepper to taste

Directions:

1. In a large bowl, combine the cucumber, tomato, red onion, and parsley.
2. In a small bowl, whisk together the olive oil, lemon juice, oregano, salt, and pepper.
3. Pour the dressing over the salad and toss to coat.
4. Serve immediately.

Nutritional information (per serving): Calories: 30, Fat: 0.5g. Carbohydrates: 7g, Fiber: 1g, Protein: 1g, Vitamin A: 30% DV, Vitamin C: 20% DV

Tips:

- For a more flavorful salad, marinate the vegetables in the dressing for 30 minutes before serving.
- You can add other vegetables to this salad, such as bell peppers, carrots, or celery.
- If you're on a strict bariatric diet, you may need to limit your intake of olive oil. You can use a calorie-free salad dressing instead.
- This salad is also a great source of potassium, which is important for maintaining healthy blood pressure.

Sugar-Free Berry Trifle

PREP TIME: 15 MINUTES | COOKING TIME: 10 MINUTES (FOR CHIA SEED PUDDING, IF USING) | TOTAL TIME: 25 MINUTES | SERVINGS: 4 INDIVIDUAL TRIFLES

Ingredients:

- 1 cup mixed berries (strawberries, blueberries, raspberries)
- 1/2 cup plain Greek yogurt (2% fat)
- 1/4 cup unsweetened almond milk
- 1/4 cup chia seeds (optional)
- 1/4 teaspoon vanilla extract
- 1/4 teaspoon ground cinnamon
- Sweetener to taste (optional, use stevia or monk fruit sweetener)

Directions:

1. Prepare the chia seed pudding (optional): If using, combine chia seeds, almond milk, vanilla extract, and cinnamon in a bowl. Stir well and let sit for 10 minutes, or until pudding thickens.
2. Assemble the trifles: Divide the berries, Greek yogurt, and chia seed pudding (if using) evenly among four serving glasses or bowls.
3. Sweeten to taste, if desired.
4. Refrigerate for at least 30 minutes before serving. This allows the flavors to meld and the chia seed pudding to fully set (if using).

Nutritional Information (per serving): Calories: 250, Carbohydrates: 20 grams (5 grams fiber), Protein: 15 grams, Fat: 5 grams

Tips:

- For a richer flavor, use full-fat Greek yogurt.
- You can substitute other berries for the ones listed in the recipe.
- Top with a sprinkle of chopped nuts or seeds for added texture and nutrients.
- If you don't have chia seeds, you can thicken the trifle with a little xanthan gum (about 1/8 teaspoon per serving).
- This trifle is best enjoyed fresh, but leftovers can be stored in the refrigerator for up to 2 days.

RECIPES FOR BIRTHDAY PARTY

Mini Caprese Skewers

PREP TIME: 10 MINUTES |COOKING TIME: 0 MINUTES | TOTAL TIME: 10 MINUTES | SERVING SIZE: 1 SKEWER (4 CHERRY TOMATOES, 4 MOZZARELLA BALLS, AND 4 BASIL LEAVES)

Ingredients:

- 8 cherry tomatoes
- 8 small mozzarella balls
- 8 fresh basil leaves
- Balsamic glaze (optional)
- Toothpicks

Dircctions:

1. Wash the cherry tomatoes and basil leaves.
2. Cut the mozzarella balls in half.
3. Assemble the skewers by threading a cherry tomato, a basil leaf, and a mozzarella ball half onto a toothpick. Repeat until all ingredients are used.
4. Drizzle with balsamic glaze, if desired.
5. Serve immediately.

Nutritional information per serving: Calories: 50, Fat: 2 grams, Carbohydrates: 5 grams, Protein: 3 grams, Fiber: 1 gram

Tlps:

- For a more flavorful appetizer, marinate the cherry tomatoes in olive oil, balsamic vinegar, and fresh herbs for 30 minutes before assembling the skewers.
- If you don't have balsamic glaze, you can use balsamic vinegar or even a little bit of olive oil.
- You can also add other ingredients to the skewers, such as cucumber slices, olives, or grilled chicken.

Chicken Lettuce Wraps

COOKING TIME: 15 MINUTES | PREP TIME: 10 MINUTES | TOTAL TIME: 25 MINUTES | SERVING SIZE: 4 LETTUCE WRAPS

Ingredients:

- 1 pound boneless, skinless chicken breast, cooked and shredded
- 1/2 cup chopped red bell pepper
- 1/4 cup chopped celery
- 1/4 cup chopped green onion
- 2 cloves garlic, minced
- 1 tablespoon soy sauce
- 1 tablespoon rice vinegar
- 1 teaspoon Sriracha (optional)
- 1/2 teaspoon sesame oil
- 1/4 cup chopped fresh cilantro
- 8 large romaine lettuce leaves

Directions:

1. In a large bowl, combine the cooked and shredded chicken, red bell pepper, celery, green onion, garlic, soy sauce, rice vinegar, Sriracha (if using), and sesame oil. Stir to combine.
2. Add the chopped cilantro and mix well.
3. Wash and dry the romaine lettuce leaves.
4. To assemble the wraps, spoon some of the chicken mixture onto each lettuce leaf. Top with your favorite toppings, such as chopped peanuts, avocado, or shredded carrots.

Nutritional Information per Serving: Calories: 250, Protein: 30g, Carbohydrates: 5g, Fiber: 2g, Fat: 10g

Tips:

- You can use ground turkey or chicken instead of chicken breast.
- If you don't have fresh cilantro, you can use 1/2 teaspoon of dried cilantro.
- For a spicier wrap, add more Sriracha or a pinch of red pepper flakes.
- These wraps can be stored in the refrigerator for up to 3 days.
- Serve these wraps with a side of brown rice or quinoa for a more complete meal.

Zucchini Pizza Bites

COOKING TIME: 15 MINUTES | PREP TIME: 10 MINUTES | TOTAL TIME: 25 MINUTES | SERVING SIZE: 12 BITES

Ingredients:

- 1 medium zucchini, thinly sliced
- 1/4 cup marinara sauce
- 1/4 cup shredded mozzarella cheese
- 1/4 cup chopped pepperoni (optional)
- 1/4 teaspoon dried oregano
- 1/4 teaspoon garlic powder
- Salt and pepper to taste

Directions:

1. Preheat oven to 400°F (200°C). Line a baking sheet with parchment paper.
2. Spread the zucchini slices on the baking sheet in a single layer. Bake for 10 minutes, or until slightly softened.
3. Flip the zucchini slices and spread each one with a thin layer of marinara sauce. Top with mozzarella cheese, pepperoni (if using), oregano, garlic powder, salt, and pepper.
4. Bake for an additional 5-7 minutes, or until the cheese is melted and bubbly.
5. Let cool slightly before serving.

Nutritional information per serving: Calories: 50, Carbohydrates: 4g, Fat: 3g, Protein: 2g, Fiber: 1g

Tips:

- You can use any type of marinara sauce you like. Just be sure to choose one that is low in sugar and sodium.
- If you don't have pepperoni, you can use any other type of topping you like, such as crumbled sausage, chopped vegetables, or even pineapple.
- These zucchini pizza bites can be stored in an airtight container in the refrigerator for up to 3 days.

Spinach and Artichoke Dip

PREP TIME: 10 MINUTES | COOKING TIME: 20 MINUTES | TOTAL TIME: 30 MINUTES | SERVING SIZE: 1/4 CUP

Ingredients:

- 1 tablespoon olive oil
- 1 onion, chopped
- 2 cloves garlic, minced
- 10 ounces frozen spinach, thawed and squeezed dry
- 1 (14.5 ounce) can artichoke hearts, drained and chopped
- 1/2 cup light ricotta cheese
- 1/4 cup fat-free Greek yogurt
- 1/4 cup grated Parmesan cheese
- 1/4 teaspoon dried oregano
- 1/4 teaspoon salt
- 1/4 teaspoon black pepper
- 1/4 cup chopped fresh parsley

Directions:

1. Heat olive oil in a large skillet over medium heat. Add onion and cook until softened, about 5 minutes.
2. Add garlic and cook for 1 minute more.
3. Stir in spinach and artichoke hearts. Cook until spinach is wilted, about 3 minutes.
4. Remove from heat and let cool slightly.
5. In a bowl, combine ricotta cheese, yogurt, Parmesan cheese, oregano, salt, and pepper. Stir in the spinach and artichoke mixture.
6. Garnish with parsley and serve with whole-wheat pita bread or crackers.

Nutritional information per serving: Calories: 150, Fat: 8 grams, Carbohydrates: 10 grams, Protein: 5 grams, Fiber: 2 grams

Tips:

- You can use fresh spinach instead of frozen, but be sure to chop it finely.
- To make the dip ahead of time, store it in the refrigerator for up to 3 days.
- If you don't have ricotta cheese, you can use cottage cheese instead.
- For a creamier dip, you can add a few tablespoons of milk or unsweetened almond milk.
- You can also serve this dip with vegetables, such as carrots, celery, or cucumbers.

Cauliflower Tater Tots

COOKING TIME: 20 MINUTES | PREP TIME: 10 MINUTES | TOTAL TIME: 30 MINUTES | SERVING SIZE: 10 TATER TOTS

Ingredients:

- 1 head of cauliflower, grated
- 1/4 cup almond flour
- 1/4 cup Parmesan cheese
- 1 egg
- 1/2 teaspoon dried oregano
- 1/4 teaspoon garlic powder
- Salt and pepper to taste

Directions:

1. Preheat oven to 400 degrees F (200 degrees C).
2. Grate the cauliflower and place it in a colander. Press down on the cauliflower to remove as much moisture as possible.
3. In a large bowl, combine the cauliflower, almond flour, Parmesan cheese, egg, oregano, garlic powder, salt, and pepper. Mix well until combined.
4. Form the mixture into small balls, about 1 inch in diameter.
5. Place the tater tots on a baking sheet lined with parchment paper.
6. Bake for 20 minutes, or until golden brown and crispy.
7. Serve immediately with your favorite dipping sauce.

Nutritional information (per serving): Calories: 50, Carbohydrates: 5 grams, Fat: 2 grams, Protein: 2 grams, Fiber: 2 grams

Tips:

- You can also use a food processor to grate the cauliflower.
- If the mixture is too wet, you can add a little more almond flour.
- You can bake the tater tots for a few minutes longer if you like them extra crispy.
- Serve the tater tots with a low-fat dipping sauce, such as ketchup, mustard, or ranch dressing.

Stuffed Mini Bell Peppers

PREP TIME: 15 MINUTES | COOK TIME: 15 MINUTES | TOTAL TIME: 30 MINUTES | SERVING SIZE: 8 MINI BELL PEPPERS (ONE PEPPER PER SERVING)

Ingredients:

- 8 mini bell peppers (any color combination you like)
- 1/2 cup ground turkey or chicken breast (lean, 90% or higher)
- 1/4 cup brown rice, cooked
- 1/4 cup chopped onion
- 1/4 cup chopped celery
- 1/4 cup chopped carrot
- 1/4 cup chopped mushrooms
- 1/4 cup chopped tomato
- 1/2 teaspoon dried oregano
- 1/4 teaspoon garlic powder
- Salt and pepper to taste

Directions:

1. Preheat oven to 375°F (190°C).
2. Wash and halve the mini bell peppers, removing the seeds and membranes.
3. In a large bowl, combine the ground turkey or chicken, cooked brown rice, onion, celery, carrot, mushrooms, tomato, oregano, garlic powder, salt, and pepper. Mix well.
4. Fill each mini bell pepper half with the stuffing mixture.
5. Place the stuffed peppers on a baking sheet lined with parchment paper.
6. Bake for 15-20 minutes, or until the peppers are tender and the filling is cooked through.

Nutritional information (per serving): Calories: 70, Fat: 1g, Carbohydrates: 5g, Fiber: 1g, Protein: 5g

Tips:

- You can use any type of ground meat you like, such as beef, lamb, or even lentil or tofu crumbles for a vegetarian option.
- Add other chopped vegetables to the stuffing, such as zucchini, spinach, or bell peppers of different colors.
- Top the stuffed peppers with a sprinkle of shredded cheese or a dollop of Greek yogurt before baking for extra flavor and protein.
- Store leftover stuffed peppers in an airtight container in the refrigerator for up to 3 days.

Bariatric-friendly Cheesecake Bites

PREP TIME: 15 MINUTES | COOKING TIME: 15 MINUTES | TOTAL TIME: 30 MINUTES | SERVING SIZE: 12 BITES

Ingredients:

- 1 cup ricotta cheese
- 1/4 cup Greek yogurt
- 1/4 cup unsweetened applesauce
- 1/4 cup almond flour
- 1/4 teaspoon vanilla extract
- 1/4 teaspoon cinnamon
- 1/4 cup sugar-free sweetener (optional)

Directions:

1. Preheat oven to 350 degrees F (175 degrees C).
2. In a large bowl, combine ricotta cheese, Greek yogurt, applesauce, almond flour, vanilla extract, and cinnamon. Mix until well combined.
3. If desired, add sugar-free sweetener to taste.
4. Spoon batter into a mini muffin tin lined with parchment paper.
5. Bake for 15 minutes, or until golden brown.
6. Let cool in the tin for at least 10 minutes before serving.

Nutritional information per serving: Calories: 100, Protein: 4 grams, Fat: 4 grams, Carbohydrates: 10 grams, Sugar: 5 grams

Tips:

- For a richer flavor, use full-fat ricotta cheese.
- You can also add other flavors to the cheesecake bites, such as chocolate chips, fruit, or nuts.
- Be sure to use sugar-free sweetener that is bariatric-friendly.
- These cheesecake bites can be stored in the refrigerator for up to 3 days.

Cucumber Rolls

PREP TIME: 10 MINUTES | COOK TIME: 5 MINUTES | TOTAL TIME: 15 MINUTES | SERVING SIZE: 1 ROLL

Ingredients:

- 1 cucumber, thinly sliced
- 1/4 cup hummus
- 1 tablespoon finely chopped red onion
- 1 tablespoon chopped fresh dill
- Pinch of salt and pepper

Directions:

1. Spread hummus evenly over the cucumber slices.
2. Top with red onion, dill, salt, and pepper.
3. Roll up the cucumber slices and enjoy!

Nutritional Information (per roll): Calories: 35, Carbohydrates: 4g, Protein: 1g, Fat: 0g, Fiber: 1g

Tips:

- For a heartier roll, use whole-wheat tortillas instead of cucumber slices.
- Add other vegetables to the rolls, such as shredded carrots, bell peppers, or spinach.
- Get creative with the toppings! Try using different types of hummus, pesto, or guacamole.

Shrimp Cocktail Shooters

PREP TIME: 10 MINUTES | COOKING TIME: 5 MINUTES (IF USING RAW SHRIMP) | TOTAL TIME: 15 MINUTES | SERVING SIZE: 1 SHOOTER

Ingredients:

- 4-5 cooked shrimp, peeled and deveined (raw can be used, see instructions)
- 1 tablespoon low-fat cocktail sauce (or homemade version, see below)
- 1 tablespoon chopped celery
- 1/2 tablespoon chopped cucumber
- 1/4 tablespoon chopped dill
- Pinch of black pepper
- Lemon wedge (optional, for garnish)

Homemade Low-Fat Cocktail Sauce:

- 1/4 cup ketchup (unsweetened)
- 1 tablespoon horseradish sauce
- 1 tablespoon lemon juice
- 1/2 teaspoon Worcestershire sauce
- Pinch of black pepper

Directions:

1. Prepare the shrimp: If using raw shrimp, bring a pot of water to a boil. Add the shrimp and cook for 3-5 minutes, or until just pink and opaque. Let cool slightly and peel and deveined.
2. Make the cocktail sauce (optional): If using store-bought, simply measure out 1 tablespoon. For the homemade version, combine all ingredients in a small bowl and stir well.
3. Assemble the shooters: Place the shrimp in the bottom of small shot glasses or martini glasses. Add the chopped celery, cucumber, and dill. Pour over the cocktail sauce until filling the glass. Add a pinch of black pepper if desired.
4. Garnish (optional): Add a lemon wedge or sprig of dill for presentation.

Nutritional Information per Serving: Calories: 70-80, Protein: 10-12g, Fat: 1-2g, Carbohydrates: 1-2g

Berry Yogurt Parfaits

PREP TIME: 5 MINUTES | COOKING TIME: 0 MINUTES | TOTAL TIME: 5 MINUTES | SERVING SIZE: 1 PARFAIT

Ingredients:

- 1/2 cup plain Greek yogurt
- 1/4 cup berries (such as blueberries, raspberries, or strawberries)
- 1/4 cup granola
- 1/4 teaspoon chia seeds

Directions:

1. In a parfait glass or bowl, layer the yogurt, berries, granola, and chia seeds.
2. Serve immediately.

Nutritional information (per serving): Calories: 250, Protein: 15 grams, Carbohydrates: 30 grams, Fat: 5 grams, Fiber: 5 grams

Tips:

- For a thicker parfait, use less yogurt.
- For a sweeter parfait, add a drizzle of honey or maple syrup.
- To make this parfait ahead of time, simply layer the ingredients in a container and store in the refrigerator overnight.
- If you're on a very restricted diet, you may need to omit the granola or use a sugar-free variety.

Dining out on a bariatric diet may be pleasurable with some careful preparation and choices. Here are some guidelines to help you make healthy selections when eating out:

Research the Menu in Advance: Many eateries post their menus online. Take the time to research the menu before you go, so you can make educated selections.

Choose Protein First: Opt for protein-rich foods such as grilled chicken, fish, lean beef, or tofu. These alternatives may help you achieve your protein requirements without excessive calories.

Avoid Fried and Breaded Foods: Steer away from fried and breaded products, since they might be heavy in calories and fat. Instead, seek for grilled, broiled, or baked choices.

Ask for Modifications: Don't hesitate to ask for adaptations to match your dietary requirements. For example, order grilled instead of fried, or ask for sauces and dressings on the side.

Watch Portion Sizes: Restaurant servings are sometimes bigger than required. Consider splitting a dish with a friend or ask for a to-go box at the beginning of the meal and pack away half.

Choose Vegetables and Fruits: Include non-starchy veggies and fresh fruits in your meal. They offer fiber, vitamins, and minerals without many calories.

Beware of Liquid Calories: Be wary of calorie-laden beverages. Opt for water, unsweetened tea, or other low-calorie choices instead of sugary drinks or alcoholic beverages.

Skip Empty Calories: Avoid empty-calorie products such as breadbaskets, chips, or excessive appetizers. Save your calories for nutrient-dense meals.

Ask for Sauces and Dressings on the Side: Request sauces and dressings on the side so you can control the quantity you use. Often, a little goes a long way.

Listen to Your Body: Pay attention to your body's hunger and fullness signs. Stop eating when you're full, and don't feel compelled to complete everything on your plate.

Be Mindful of Hidden Sugars: Watch out for hidden sugars in sauces, dressings, and marinades. Choose foods with low added sugars.

Plan for Dessert: If you want dessert, try sharing it or settle for a small, lighter choice. Fresh fruit or a small amount of sorbet may be filling without overdoing it.

Portion Control Strategies

Portion management is critical for persons following a bariatric diet, helping limit calorie intake and assist in weight reduction or maintenance. Here are some helpful ways to manage portions:

Use Smaller Plates and Bowls: Downsizing your tableware might provide the appearance of greater quantities. It fools the mind into feeling content with less food.

Practice the Plate Method: Divide your meal into sections: half for non-starchy veggies, a quarter for lean protein, and a quarter for a complex carbohydrate. This visually balanced method helps manage portions.

Pre-Portion Snacks: Instead of eating straight from a bag or container, pre-portion food into little containers or baggies. This reduces thoughtless overeating.

Mindful Eating: Pay attention to each mouthful by eating carefully and appreciating the tastes. This helps your body to detect fullness, minimizing the probability of overeating.

Listen to Hunger Cues: Eat when you're hungry and quit when you're content. Avoid eating out of boredom or as a reaction to emotions.

Measure and Weigh Foods: Use measuring cups, a food scale, or visual comparisons to get acquainted with acceptable portion amounts. This helps you build a better grasp of portion control.

Order or Cook Small Portions: When dining out, consider ordering appetizer-sized portions or sharing a dish with someone. When cooking at home, prepare fewer quantities to minimize leftovers enticing you to overeat.

Limit Liquid Calories: Be mindful of high-calorie beverages. Choose water or other low-calorie options to prevent consuming excessive calories in liquid form.

Pack Leftovers Immediately: If you're at a restaurant or cooking at home, pack away leftovers right after serving to avoid going back for seconds.

Use Your Hand as a Guide: Your hand can be a handy tool for estimating portion sizes. For example, a serving of protein is about the size of your palm, a serving of vegetables is about the size of your fist, and a serving of fats is about the size of your thumb.

Avoid Buffets and All-You-Can-Eat Options: Buffets can be challenging for portion control. If possible, choose restaurants with single-serving options or order a la carte.

Be Selective at Events: When attending events with a variety of food options, survey the offerings before deciding what to eat. Choose smaller portions of your favorite items.

Plan and Log Meals: Planning your meals and logging your food can help you stay accountable and make more conscious choices about portion sizes.

Eat Balanced Meals: Include a balance of macronutrients (protein, carbohydrates, and fats) in your meals. This can enhance satiety and help you avoid overeating.

Communicating Dietary Needs

Effectively communicating your dietary needs when dining out is crucial to ensure that your meals align with your bariatric diet. Here are some tips on how to communicate your dietary needs to restaurant staff:

Be clear and specific: Clearly express your dietary restrictions and needs. Specify if you need low-fat, low-carb, high-protein, or specific portion sizes.

Ask Questions: Don't hesitate to ask questions about the menu items. Inquire about ingredients, cooking methods, and possible substitutions to make informed choices.

Use Positive Language: Positively frame your requests. Instead of saying what you can't have, focus on what you can eat. For example, "I'm looking for a lean protein option, such as grilled chicken or fish."

Request Modifications: Most restaurants are willing to accommodate dietary preferences. Ask for modifications like grilled instead of fried, sauce on the side, or substituting certain ingredients.

Express the Importance of Your Needs: If your dietary needs are critical for health reasons, politely convey this to the restaurant staff. Emphasize the importance of adhering to your specific requirements.

Use Allergen Terminology: If applicable, use allergy-related terms to stress the seriousness of your dietary needs. For instance, saying you have a gluten sensitivity may convey the importance more effectively.

Be Prepared to Educate: Some staff may not be familiar with bariatric diets. Be prepared to provide a brief explanation of your dietary needs and what types of foods are suitable for you.

Check for Hidden Ingredients: Ask about hidden ingredients, such as added sugars, sauces, or dressings. These can significantly impact the nutritional content of a dish.

Speak directly to the Chef: If you have specific and detailed dietary needs, consider asking to speak directly to the chef. They can often provide more accurate information about ingredients and preparation methods.

Express Appreciation: Show gratitude when the staff accommodates your requests. A positive and appreciative attitude can go a long way in ensuring a pleasant dining experience.

Use Online Resources: Some restaurants provide nutritional information online. Check their website or contact them in advance to gather information about the menu.

Consider Local or Health-Conscious Restaurants: Choose restaurants that are known for offering healthier options or that cater to specific dietary needs. These establishments may be more accustomed to accommodating special requests.

Remember that effective communication is key to a successful dining experience. Don't be afraid to advocate for your needs, and be patient and polite while interacting with restaurant staff. Most establishments are willing to work with customers to ensure a positive and enjoyable dining experience.

Dealing with Food Intolerances

Dealing with food intolerances after bariatric surgery is common and can present challenges as your digestive system adjusts to changes. Here are some common challenges related to food intolerances post-bariatric surgery and potential solutions:

CHALLENGES:

Difficulty Digesting Certain Foods: After surgery, some individuals may struggle to digest certain foods, leading to discomfort, nausea, or vomiting.

Food Aversions: Changes in taste and smell can result in food aversions, making it challenging to consume specific foods.

Reactive Hypoglycemia: Some individuals may experience reactive hypoglycemia, where blood sugar levels drop rapidly after eating, leading to symptoms like shakiness, sweating, and dizziness.

Dumping Syndrome: Rapid gastric emptying, known as dumping syndrome, can occur after consuming high-sugar or high-fat foods, leading to symptoms such as nausea, sweating, and diarrhea.

SOLUTIONS:

Gradual Introduction of Foods: Slowly reintroduce new foods to gauge tolerance. Start with small amounts and monitor your body's response.

Focus on Protein: Prioritize protein-rich foods as they are essential for muscle maintenance and can be better-tolerated post-surgery.

Chew Thoroughly: Chew food thoroughly to aid digestion. This is particularly important after bariatric surgery when the stomach capacity is reduced.

Hydration: Stay hydrated, but avoid drinking large amounts with meals, as it can contribute to discomfort. Sip water between meals.

Identify Trigger Foods: Keep a food diary to identify trigger foods that cause discomfort or adverse reactions. This can help you tailor your diet to avoid problematic items.

Supplementation: If certain foods are difficult to tolerate, consider supplementation to ensure you're meeting nutritional needs. Consult with a dietitian for personalized recommendations.

Regular Follow-Ups: Attend regular follow-up appointments with your healthcare team, including dietitians, to discuss any challenges and receive guidance on managing food intolerances.

Meal Timing: Optimize meal timing to prevent reactive hypoglycemia. Eat smaller, balanced meals at regular intervals throughout the day.

Avoid Trigger Foods: Identify and avoid foods that trigger dumping syndrome, such as high-sugar and high-fat items. Opt for nutrient-dense, whole foods instead.

Cooking Methods: Choose gentle cooking methods like baking, steaming, or grilling. Avoid heavy frying, as it may be harder to digest.

Mindful Eating: Practice mindful eating by paying attention to hunger and fullness cues. Avoid distractions while eating to promote better digestion.

Support Groups: Join bariatric support groups to share experiences and strategies with others who have undergone similar surgeries.

OVERCOMING PLATEAUS

Experiencing plateaus in weight loss is not uncommon, especially after bariatric surgery. Plateaus can be frustrating, but there are strategies to overcome them and continue progressing towards your weight loss goals. Here are some tips:

Reevaluate Your Diet: Take a serious look at your existing eating habits. Are there any hidden calories or unwise dietary choices that can hurt your progress? Consider talking with a qualified dietitian to examine and change your dietary plan.

Monitor Portion Sizes: Ensure you are exercising portion control properly. It's common for portion sizes to sneak up over time, so be conscious of what and how much you are consuming.

Check for Hidden Calories: Be mindful of additional sweets, high-calorie sauces, and liquid calories. Even tiny quantities may add up, influencing your total calorie consumption.

Stay Hydrated: Proper hydration is vital for general health and may also assist in weight reduction. Drink water throughout the day and avoid sugary drinks.

Review Physical Activity: Evaluate your workout routine. Are you integrating both cardiovascular workouts and strength training? Adding diversity to your routines might help break past a rut.

Adjust Caloric Intake: As your body changes post-surgery, your calorie demands may also shift. Consult with your healthcare provider to decide whether a modification in your calorie intake is required.

Increase Physical Activity Intensity: If you've been regularly exercising, try increasing the intensity of your sessions. This might be via longer workouts, greater intensity intervals, or introducing new activities.

Break up Meals: Instead of three big meals, try splitting them into smaller, more regular meals. This may help control blood sugar levels and enhance your metabolism.

Manage Stress: High-stress levels might hinder weight loss. Practice stress-reducing activities such as mindfulness, yoga, or deep breathing techniques.

Sleep Quality: Ensure you are receiving adequate and quality sleep. Lack of sleep might interfere with weight reduction attempts.

Set Realistic Goals: Reevaluate your weight reduction objectives. Set reasonable, attainable aims that fit with your body's reaction to the operation.

Consider Medical Evaluation: If you've tried several tactics and still suffer a plateau, contact your healthcare provider. There can be underlying causes that need to be addressed.

Celebrate Non-Scale Victories: Focus on non-scale successes, such as more energy, higher exercise levels, and better overall health. Sometimes, the scale doesn't represent the wonderful improvements in your body.

Stay Patient and Persistent: Weight reduction plateaus are a frequent aspect of the process. Keep patient, keep focused, and remain persistent. Consistency is crucial to breaking through plateaus.

Emotional Eating Coping Strategies

Emotional eating is a typical difficulty, and establishing coping methods is vital for maintaining a good relationship with food, particularly after bariatric surgery. Here are some techniques to assist in controlling emotional eating:

Identify Triggers: Pay attention to events or feelings that induce emotional eating. Keep a notebook to chronicle what you're experiencing when the impulse to eat emotionally occurs.

Find Alternative Coping Mechanisms: Replace emotional eating with better-coping techniques such as deep breathing, meditation, exercise, writing, or talking to a friend.

Create a Support System: Share your emotions with friends, relatives, or a support group. Having a solid support system may give emotional support and understanding.

Mindful Eating: Practice mindful eating by paying attention to the flavor, texture, and fragrance of your meal. Eat without interruptions, appreciating each mouthful.

Develop Healthy Habits: Establish healthy routines that don't require eating, like taking a stroll, reading a book, or indulging in a pastime.

Delay Eating: If you sense the temptation to emotionally eat, wait for the activity for a defined duration (e.g., 10 minutes). Use this time to examine if you are hungry or whether the impulse to eat is emotional.

Positive Affirmations: Use positive affirmations to increase your mood and self-esteem. Remind yourself of your successes, strengths, and motivations for pursuing bariatric surgery.

Seek Professional Help: If emotional eating is chronic and tough to manage on your own, consider seeking the support of a therapist or counselor who specializes in eating disorders or emotional well-being.

Build Resilience: Work on strengthening emotional resilience by establishing coping skills and techniques to manage stress and tough emotions without resorting to food.

Create a Relaxation Routine: Establish a relaxation regimen that helps you unwind and manage stress. This might include things like taking a warm bath, doing yoga or listening to relaxing music.

Keep Healthy Snacks Available: Stock your house with healthful snacks that are matched with your bariatric diet. When the need to eat comes, go for healthful choices.

Stay Hydrated: Drink water throughout the day. Sometimes, sensations of hunger might be confused for dehydration.

Set Realistic Goals: Set manageable and realistic objectives for your weight reduction journey. Unrealistic expectations might lead to anger and emotional eating.

Celebrate Non-Food Achievements: Celebrate successes that have nothing to do with eating. Recognize and reward yourself for attaining milestones, whether they are connected to your health, personal progress, or successes at work.

Be Kind to Yourself: Practice self-compassion. Understand that everyone has times of emotional eating, and it's acceptable. Be nice to yourself, learn from the experience, and go on.

Staying active and concentrating on general well-being are key components of a bariatric journey. Here are some exercise and wellness suggestions to maintain your health following bariatric surgery:

FITNESS TIPS:

Start Slowly: Begin with low-impact activities and progressively build intensity. Walking is a fantastic beginning place, and as your fitness level increases, you may try additional sports like swimming or cycling.

Include Strength Training: Incorporate strength training activities to increase and maintain muscular mass. Resistance exercise may aid with toning and raising metabolism.

Work with a Professional: Consult with a fitness expert or physical therapist who has experience dealing with clients who have had bariatric surgery. They may give specific workout suggestions based on your demands and restrictions.

Choose Activities You Enjoy: Find things you like to make exercise a sustainable part of your routine. Whether it's dancing, hiking, or group fitness programs, having fun may enhance your motivation.

Stay Consistent: Consistency is crucial. Aim for frequent, moderate activity throughout the week rather than random intensive exercises. This technique is more sustainable and helpful for long-term health.

Listen to Your Body: Pay attention to how your body reacts to exercise. If you encounter pain or discomfort, alter the exercise or check with a healthcare practitioner.

Mix Cardio and Strength Training: A well-rounded fitness plan involves both aerobic workouts (such as walking, running, or swimming) and strength training. This combo enhances general fitness and weight control.

Set Realistic Goals: Establish attainable fitness objectives. Start with minor goals and progressively raise the intensity or length of your exercises as your strength and endurance develop.

WELLNESS TIPS:

Stay Hydrated: Adequate hydration is vital for general health and may promote weight reduction. Drink water throughout the day, particularly before and after activity.

Prioritize Nutrition: Follow your bariatric diet plan to ensure you're receiving the required nutrients for recovery and good health. Consult with a nutritionist to make any required modifications depending on your activity level.

Get Sufficient Sleep: Aim for 7-9 hours of decent sleep each night. Sleep is vital for recuperation, metabolism, and general well-being.

Manage Stress: Practice stress-management strategies such as meditation, deep breathing, or yoga. Chronic stress may significantly influence both physical and mental health.

Connect with Support Groups: Join bariatric support organizations or communities. Connecting with individuals who have encountered similar circumstances may give essential support, inspiration, and insights.

Regular Follow-ups: Attend frequent follow-up meetings with your healthcare team, including your surgeon, dietician, and fitness specialists. Regular check-ins may assist in tracking your development and resolve any problems.

Practice Mindful Eating: Be cautious of your dietary habits. Pay attention to hunger and fullness indicators, and minimize distractions when eating.

Celebrate Non-Scale Victories: Acknowledge and appreciate victories outside the scale, such as greater energy, higher fitness levels, and good changes in mood.

Incorporating Exercise into Your Routine

Consult with Your Healthcare Team: Before beginning any exercise program, check with your healthcare team, including your surgeon and a fitness expert. They may give advice based on your individual health state and surgery history.

Start slow and gradual: Begin with low-impact exercises and develop gradually. Walking is a wonderful first exercise. As your fitness level increases, you may integrate more strenuous activities.

Choose Activities You Enjoy: Find workouts that you love. Whether it's swimming, dancing, cycling, or yoga, picking activities you enjoy enhances the probability that you'll keep with them.

Establish a Routine: Set a steady workout plan. Schedule your exercises at a time that fits your lifestyle, whether it's in the morning, around lunch, or in the evening.

Mix Cardio and Strength Training: A well-rounded fitness plan involves both aerobic workouts (e.g., walking, running, swimming) and strength training. Strength training is vital for preserving muscle mass, particularly after bariatric surgery.

Use Short Bouts of Exercise: Break your activity into shorter, more doable periods throughout the day. Even 10-15 minutes of exercise numerous times a day might be useful.

Include Everyday Activities: Incorporate physical exercise into your everyday life. Take the stairs instead of the elevator, walk or bike instead of driving small distances, and find chances to exercise throughout the day.

Set Realistic Goals: Establish attainable fitness objectives. Start with minor goals and progressively raise the intensity or length of your exercises as your strength and endurance develop.

Use Fitness Apps or Wearable's: Consider utilizing fitness apps or wearable's to measure your progress. Monitoring your steps, exercises, and other data may give you motivation and a feeling of success.

Join Group Classes or Activities: Participate in group fitness courses or activities. This may give social support, drive, and a feeling of community.

Listen to Your Body: Pay attention to how your body reacts to exercise. If you suffer pain, dizziness, or discomfort, reduce the activity or talk with your healthcare staff.

Stay Hydrated: Drink water before, during, and after exercise to keep hydrated. Adequate hydration is vital for general health.

Warm-up and Cool Down: Always warm up before activity and cool down afterward. This helps avoid injuries and increases flexibility.

Celebrate Progress: Celebrate your victories along the way. Whether it's hitting a specific step count, lifting a higher weight, or finishing a program, recognize your success.

Be Consistent: Consistency is crucial to obtaining long-term effects from exercise. Make physical exercise a regular part of your routine to enjoy the full rewards.

Mindful Eating Practices

Mindful eating is a discipline that entails paying full attention to the experience of eating, relishing each mouthful, and being completely present in the moment. This method may be especially effective following bariatric surgery to establish good eating habits and assist in long-term weight maintenance. Here are some mindful eating habits to add to your routine:

Eat Without Distractions: Avoid eating in front of the TV, computer, or while looking through your phone. Create a designated, calm location for meals to completely concentrate on your cuisine.

Engage Your Senses: Take a minute to savor the colors, textures, and fragrances of your cuisine. Engage your senses completely in the dining experience.

Chew Thoroughly: Chew your meal slowly and completely. This not only assists digestion but also lets you appreciate the tastes and textures of each meal.

Savor Each Bite: Pause between mouthfuls and relish the flavor of your meal. Enjoy the experience rather than racing through the meal.

Listen to Hunger Cues: Tune in to your body's hunger and fullness signs. Eat when you're hungry and quit when you're full, avoiding overeating.

Be Mindful of Portion Sizes: Pay attention to portion sizes and avoid eating past the point of fullness. Use smaller dishes and bowls to aid with portion management.

Eat with Intention: Before eating, take a minute to establish an intention for your meal. Consider why you're eating and what you intend to gain from the experience.

Pause between Bites: Put your utensils down between eating. This simple gesture promotes a slower pace and enables you to concentrate on the process of eating.

Identify Emotional Eating Triggers: Be conscious of emotional eating triggers. If you find yourself grabbing food in reaction to emotions, stop and consider alternate strategies to deal with those sensations.

Appreciate Your Food's Journey: Consider the path your food went to reach your plate. Acknowledge the labor required in cultivating, harvesting, and preparing the food.

Express Gratitude: Take time to express thanks for your meal. Reflect on the sustenance it gives and the labor that went into making it.

Recognize Fullness: Pay attention to the indicators of fullness, such as a contented sensation or a slower rate of eating. Stop eating when you feel pleasantly full.

Enjoy the Company: If you're eating with others, enjoy the company and conversation. Engage in good and thoughtful relationships rather than focus primarily on the meal.

Practice Moderation: Embrace an attitude of moderation. Allow yourself to enjoy a range of meals in moderation rather than developing restricted eating habits.

Reflect on Food Choices: After eating, think about how the meal made you feel physically and emotionally. Use this knowledge to make thoughtful decisions in the future.

Building a Supportive Community

Building a supporting group is vital for anybody facing the obstacles of bariatric surgery and post-surgical life. A solid support system may give encouragement, understanding, and practical counsel. Here are some strategies for developing a supportive community:

Join Bariatric Support Groups: Look for local or online bariatric support groups. These communities frequently comprise of people who have encountered similar situations and may give significant insights, advice, and emotional support.

Attend Regular Support Group Meetings: Attend frequent support group meetings to keep connected with others on a similar path. Share your experiences, listen to others, and gain from the collective knowledge of the community.

Engage in Online Communities: Explore internet forums, social media groups, or specialized venues for bariatric surgery patients. Participate in conversations, ask questions, and share your own experiences.

Connect with Your Healthcare Team: Foster a close relationship with your healthcare team, including your surgeon, dietician, and mental health providers. Regular check-ins and follow-ups may give continuing assistance and direction.

Involve Family and Friends: Educate your family and friends about your bariatric journey. Share your objectives, difficulties, and how they can help you. Having a good support system at home is vital.

Encourage Open Communication: Create an atmosphere where free communication is encouraged. Be honest about your needs and emotions, and let people know how they can best help you.

Share Achievements and Challenges: Celebrate your victories, no matter how tiny, with your support community. Similarly, don't hesitate to discuss your problems. This openness develops a feeling of understanding and connection.

Participate in Wellness Activities Together: Engage in healthy activities with your support community. This might include group fitness sessions, food demos, or other health-focused activities.

Provide Mutual Support: Offer help to people in your community. Sometimes, being present for others may boost your feeling of purpose and resilience.

Create a Positive Environment: Foster a good and encouraging community environment. Encourage one another, and concentrate on solutions and encouragement rather than lingering on issues.

Educate yourself and others: Stay informed about bariatric surgery and related subjects. Educate yourself and others to refute falsehoods and foster understanding.

Volunteer for Support Activities: Volunteer to assist in planning or participate in support activities. Being actively engaged in the community may develop your ties and contribute to a feeling of belonging.

Respect Diversity of Experiences: Recognize that everyone's bariatric journey is unique. Respect and celebrate the variety of experiences within your community.

Attend Events and Workshops: Attend bariatric-related activities, seminars, or conferences. These meetings allow opportunity to interact with others, learn from professionals, and remain inspired.

Seek Professional Support: If required, seek the counsel of mental health experts who specialize in bariatric surgery. Therapy or counseling may be a great resource for managing the emotional parts of the experience.

Remember, developing a supportive community is a continuous effort. Be patient, open-minded, and proactive in seeking and offering help. Surrounding oneself with a supportive and understanding group may dramatically increase your general well-being during and after your bariatric journey.

FREQUENTLY ASKED QUESTIONS

What is bariatric surgery?

Bariatric surgery is a surgical treatment used to promote weight reduction by lowering the quantity of food the stomach can retain, reducing nutritional absorption, or both.

What are the various forms of bariatric surgery?

Common types include gastric bypass, sleeve gastrectomy, gastric banding, and biliopancreatic diversion with duodenal switch.

Why is a particular diet essential after bariatric surgery?

The digestive system experiences major changes following surgery, and a particular diet offers sufficient nourishment while aiding weight reduction.

What is the post-bariatric surgery diet progression?

Typically, it begins with clear liquids, proceeds to full liquids, then to puree and soft meals, and then to a normal diet over many weeks.

How does the bariatric diet differ from other diets?

The bariatric diet is particularly formulated to fit the dietary demands and limits of persons who have had weight reduction surgery.

What are the standards for protein consumption post-bariatric surgery?

Protein is necessary for mending and maintaining muscular mass. Guidelines frequently encourage a high-protein diet, including sources like lean meats, dairy, and plant-based proteins.

How can I guarantee I'm receiving adequate vitamins and minerals?

Supplementation is typically essential post-bariatric surgery. Regular blood tests help check nutritional levels, and supplements may include vitamins B12, D, and iron.

Can I consume alcohol after bariatric surgery?

Alcohol metabolism may be impacted post-surgery, and it's typically suggested to reduce alcohol consumption. Consult with your healthcare team for specific advice.

How does exercise play into a bariatric lifestyle?

Exercise is crucial for general health, weight control, and muscle upkeep. It is frequently suggested as part of a post-bariatric lifestyle.

How can I handle emotional eating after surgery?

Emotional eating may be handled by mindful eating practices, receiving help from a therapist, and creating alternate coping methods.

What are the keys to long-term success following bariatric surgery?

Long-term success entails sticking to dietary rules, remaining physically active, attending frequent check-ups, and maintaining a supportive lifestyle.

Can I recover weight after bariatric surgery?

Weight regain is possible, but dedication to a nutritious diet, frequent exercise, and continued support may help avoid it.

How can I locate a bariatric support group?

Look for local or online support groups via hospitals, clinics, or internet platforms where folks exchange experiences and provide encouragement.

Can I dine out with friends and family after surgery?

Yes, but making sensible eating choices is key. Choose fewer servings, concentrate on protein, and avoid high-calorie or sugary alternatives.

Can I still enjoy my favorite meals after bariatric surgery?

Moderation is crucial. While certain meals may need to be restricted, modest servings of decadent delights may still be eaten sometimes.

How can I handle portion control effectively?

Use smaller plates, eat slowly, and heed your body's hunger and fullness signals. This helps avoid overeating.

Are there certain foods to avoid following bariatric surgery?

High-calorie, high-sugar, and high-fat foods should be minimized. Carbonated drinks and tough foods may also be hard to digest.

How do I tackle dietary intolerances post-bariatric surgery?

Keep a food journal to identify trigger foods, introduce new meals gradually, and consider supplementing if particular foods are tough to stomach.

What is dumping syndrome, and how may it be avoided?

Dumping syndrome is a group of symptoms after consuming high-sugar or high-fat meals. To avoid it, focus on a balanced diet, limit sugary foods, and eat smaller, more frequent meals.

How can I incorporate exercise into my routine after surgery?

Start cautiously with low-impact workouts and progressively build intensity. Consult with your healthcare provider and discover things you love to keep motivated.

How do I deal with emotional eating?

Practice mindful eating, identify emotional triggers, seek support from a therapist, and develop alternative coping strategies such as deep breathing or engaging in hobbies.

What should I do if I hit a weight loss plateau?

Reevaluate your diet, monitor portion sizes, check for hidden calories, increase physical activity intensity, and consider consulting with your healthcare team for personalized guidance.

Are non-scale victories important in bariatric success?

Yes, celebrating non-scale victories, such as increased energy, improved fitness, and positive lifestyle changes, is crucial for long-term motivation and success.

How do I communicate my dietary needs when dining out?

Call ahead, ask for menu modifications, choose protein-rich options, and communicate your needs to the waiter. Planning can make dining out enjoyable and stress-free.

What role does a supportive community play in post-bariatric success?

A supportive community provides encouragement, understanding, and shared experiences. Joining support groups and connecting with others can enhance your bariatric journey.

GLOSSARY

Anastomosis: The surgical connection of two structures, generally alluding to the link between the stomach and the small intestine in bariatric surgery.

Bariatric Surgery: Surgical treatments are done on the stomach or intestines to stimulate weight reduction, such as gastric bypass, sleeve gastrectomy, or gastric banding.

BMI (Body Mass Index): A measure of body fat based on height and weight. It is typically used to define persons as underweight, normal weight, overweight, or obese.

Calorie Density: The quantity of calories in a particular volume of food. Bariatric diets frequently concentrate on nutrient-dense, low-calorie meals to help weight reduction.

Carbohydrates: One of the three macronutrients, along with protein and fat. Carbohydrates are a key source of energy and comprise sugars, starches, and fiber.

Dumping Syndrome: A set of symptoms, including nausea and diarrhea that may occur after consuming high-sugar or high-fat meals after some bariatric procedures.

Eating Window: The exact time of the day when folks have their meals. Some bariatric diets may propose particular eating windows.

Fiber: A form of carbohydrate that is not completely digested by the body. Fiber is vital for digestive health and may contribute to a sensation of fullness.

Gastric Bypass: A form of bariatric surgery that includes constructing a tiny stomach pouch and rerouting the small intestine to bypass a section of it.

Hydration: The process of maintaining appropriate fluid levels in the body. Staying hydrated is vital for general health and post-bariatric surgery recovery.

Malabsorption: The reduced absorption of nutrients by the digestive tract, is commonly a consequence of certain bariatric procedures.

Protein: A macronutrient necessary for creating and repairing tissues. Bariatric diets highlight the significance of getting adequate protein.

Restriction: The decrease of stomach size or change of the digestive system to restrict food intake, often done via bariatric surgery.

Sleeve Gastrectomy: A bariatric surgery that involves removing a part of the stomach to produce a smaller, banana-shaped stomach pouch.

Stapling: A surgical method used in bariatric surgery to form partitions or seal off sections of the stomach or intestines.

Total Daily Allowance (TDA): The recommended daily intake of calories and nutrients for those following a bariatric diet.

Dumping Syndrome: A set of symptoms, including nausea and diarrhea that may occur after consuming high-sugar or high-fat meals after some bariatric procedures.

Water Soluble Vitamins: Vitamins that dissolve in water, include vitamin C and B-complex vitamins. These vitamins are necessary for many body activities.

This vocabulary gives a starting point, and you may adjust it further depending on the unique theme and content of your bariatric diet cookbook. Adding brief and clear definitions would increase the overall user experience for readers.

www.ingramcontent.com/pod-product-compliance
Lightning Source LLC
Chambersburg PA
CBHW080926260726
48661CB00010B/3811